"The conduct of right and good relationships between human being must ultimately concern every authentic ethical theory. Bergum and Dossetor offer an insightful analysis of the moral status of relationships that should interest professional and general readers alike."

Edmund D. Pellegrino, MD
Professor Emeritus of Medicine and Medical Ethics
Georgetown University Medical Center

"This landmark work introduces an approach to healthcare ethics for our times. Bergum (Nursing) and Dossetor (Medicine) present the core elements of relational ethics in an immediate, accessible, and inspiring way by gathering the reader around genuine stories, bringing this ethic to life. Clinicians engaging with relational ethics quickly realize its value. As one clinician told me, 'I've practiced in healthcare for 23 years and I never really *got* ethics. I get this!'"

Wendy Austin, PhD
Professor Emeritus
Canada Research Chair, Relational Ethics in Health Care (2003-2013)
University of Alberta

"Relational ethics supports each nurse's instinctive moral compass to think and act in terms of self-in-relation, creating healing environments that support the development of unique and diverse human beings. As Bergum and Dossetor suggest, "we breathe in ethical tension and breathe out ethical action. ... In the immediacy of the moment we replace objectivity with dialogue, and we replace principles with relationship." This enlightening book inspires lively student conversations and many *aha* moments."

Martha Mathews Libster, PhD, MSN, PMH-CNS
Director, Nursing Academic Partnership Design
Rogers Behavioral Health
Founding Director, Self-care Institute at Golden Apple Healing Arts

Relational Ethics

The Full Meaning of Respect

Relational Ethics

The Full Meaning of Respect

Vangie Bergum
and John Dossetor

Ansuz Media
Courtenay, BC

Figure 1, in chapter 3, originally appeared in Lesley Paulette, "A Choice
for Kaila," *Humane Medicine* 9, no. 1 (1993): 13-7, p. 14, and is used with the
kind permission of Multimed. © 1993 Multimed. All rights reserved.

2020 Reprint

Relational Ethics: The Full Meaning of Respect, first published in 2005, is reprinted in response to health care professionals' expressed wish to have a book that emphasizes our relational commitments to one another. The relational approach to ethical decision-making brings knowledge back to our life experience in order to discover how to act and how to be with each other.

The 2020 global pandemic and the demonstrations against systemic racism show the vitality of a relational ethic. Both the unruly novel coronavirus and ever-present racism demonstrate that all people, irrespective of race, gender, age, ethnicity, sexual orientation, culture, religion, or ability are interdependent and therefore impacted. In such an interconnected world respect for one another is our needed ethical commitment.

Foundational knowledge for a relational ethic, found in this book, is an action ethic experienced in issues of everyday life. A relational ethic emphasizes mutual respect, engagement with each other, the use of knowledge of mind and body, and the creation of an environment where these relational elements can flourish. Deep respect for one another is at the heart of treatments during the pandemic, as well as in our actions to achieve a society where all can live in freedom and equality.

This reprint of *Relational Ethics: The Full Meaning of Respect* honours the memory of Dr. John Beamish Dossetor (July 19, 1925 - April 6, 2020). John Dossetor with his wise council showed respect for others, whether patients, students, clinicians, academics, staff or public. He was a thoughtful and gracious man. An inspiration. He is missed.

Vangie Bergum, PhD
Professor Emeritus
University of Alberta

Contents

In memory of Sandra McKinnon (1954-2000),
a member of the Interdisciplinary Research Group
whose practice embodied all that is relational ethics.

Acknowledgments

One of the truly wonderful outcomes of the Relational Ethics Research Project has been the continuing interest and commitment of the individuals associated with the project. While the first phase of the project, which began in 1994, is the focus of this book, the research continued with a second phase that focused on mental health, genetic counseling, and relations between healthcare providers. The continuing research, which will result in other publications, kept the project alive and exciting for this extended period—and it was hard to be absolutely clear which phase we were in. All participants of the research, those in the role of investigators, members of the Interdisciplinary Research Group (IRG, listed in appendix A), graduate and undergraduate research assistants, and graduate students who explored ideas in courses, are all a part of the success of this project. It is hard to acknowledge the value that each conversation, each feedback on the written word, and each discussion of articles and lectures had for the interpretative work presented here.

We do need to identify particular individuals who kept reminding us of our task and the need to complete the text. These people believed that a written text would give further opportunity to develop and clarify the need for a relational ethic and what it means to healthcare professionals in practice. Our debt of gratitude goes to Sandra MacPhail, our project director, whose clear commitment to the work held the project together and kept us all informed about the various ongoing activities. We want to give Sandy a special acknowledgment for her contribution. Colleagues, in roles of co-investigators in Phase 2, Wendy Austin, Stephen Bamforth, Susan James, and Marion Briggs, collaborated in the analysis of the research, development of the themes, and critique of the written text. We thank these individuals for their vital contributions. Many of our readers included graduate students who have now finished their studies, such as Simon Nuttgens, Marilyn Evans, Eleanor Stewart, Dianne Godkin, Diane Desjardins, Bernie Pauly, Patricia Marck, Anna Santos Salas, Lela Zimmer, Diane Gamble, and Bashir Jiwani. All commented, discussed, and challenged the ideas presented here. Undergraduate summer students were also part of the project, and we thank Marika Warren, Kristin Warner, and Donna King. Dianne Godkin is also thanked for her technical and editorial assistance in the publication of the text.

For a number of years, graduate students in courses taught by Vangie Bergum were encouraged to consider the usefulness of a relational ethic in their own practice—whether as nurses, physicians, philosophers, clergy, pastoral counselors, or teachers. Margaret Shone, a member of the IRG, has taken the ideas into the practice of law, especially family law, and we are excited about her projects. Sally Gadow was an early consultant in the project, and we are grateful to her for her generous time commitment and her exceptional guidance. We also wish to thank Brenda Cameron for her careful reading of the completed text and sharing her valuable insights.

Of course, the research project and the book could not have been begun without the funding support of the Social Sciences and Humanities Research Council of Canada. The John Dossetor Health Ethics Centre at the University of Alberta provided a lovely, comfortable environment in which to hold our research meetings. Many hours were spent in the Dossetor Ethics Centre in dialogue about our ethical commitments to ourselves and to each other. Our faculty colleagues, particularly Paul Byrne, as well as Edna Cunningham Liley and Eileen Crookes, are thanked for their generous enthusiasm for the project and for the work it brought to each of them.

Our families, especially our spouses, Brault Kelpin and Margaret Dossetor, need to be acknowledged for their support of the research project itself (those many Saturday mornings) and for the writing (the seemingly endless hours on evenings and weekends). We thank them.

Leslie LeBlanc, president of University Publishing Group, has been an excellent editor. We appreciate her ongoing commitment in bringing this book to completion. Dr. Solomon Benatar is thanked for his commentary, which is found in the Foreword.

While we have benefited greatly, all the support we received, from individuals, from funding agencies, and from institutions, we take full responsibility for the ideas that are presented here.

Vangie Bergum
John Dossetor

Foreword

Medicine and the provision of healthcare have changed profoundly over the past 50 years. Major advances in scientific knowledge have been translated into highly specialized practical progress in supporting and prolonging life through the application of advanced technology by an ever-enlarging medical team. Market forces and market values increasingly dominate life, and the provision of healthcare and the conduct of medical research have become incrementally commercialized. Growth of bureaucracy has added layers of control with a view to standardizing research and practice and making practitioners accountable. Professionalism has come under fire and, to a considerable extent, has been modified and somewhat eclipsed under the influence of market and bureaucratic forces.

The idea of what medical ethics is about is also changing. A set of long-held and unquestioned professionally determined values that were never openly taught, but were propagated through example and social expectations, has been replaced by the formal discipline of bioethics, significantly influenced by conceptual analyses provided by philosophers, the empirical work of social scientists, and contributions from law. A reasoned, evidence-based, and due process approach to ethical decision making is now encouraged. Guidelines and rules beginning with the *Nuremberg Code* have proliferated, and bioethics has become a field of activity occupied by a range of scholars from a variety of academic backgrounds. It has also become a contested terrain on which battles have raged about concepts, values, practices, and about how ethics should be taught and applied.

While ethics is a branch of philosophy that critically examines what distinguishes right and good from wrong and bad, it can be argued that the cognitive approach does little to ensure moral behavior. Philosophers respond to such criticism with the claim that their role is to clarify what is right and good, and to provide justification for their conclusions, not to teach people to be more moral. As such, ethics education may be seen to be predominantly about acquiring deeper knowledge of ethics and not about exhortation to exemplary moral action, although it is hoped that improved moral behavior will be promoted by knowing what is the right and good thing to do—and seeing how decisions are made and implemented in practice.

The scope and pattern of the bioethics endeavor has been considerably shaped by the notion that the world is made up of reflective, autonomous, self-determining individuals whose right to make choices for themselves is the most sacrosanct value in political life and in healthcare. The value of community and of relationships has been undervalued, and a dispassionate world of strangers has been constructed in which we are primarily responsible only for ourselves.

This book is about how to rectify such alienation by refocusing on relationships—what relationships are about, how they are created, what they mean, and how they are sustained. The authors make the justifiable assertion that human flourishing is enhanced by healthy and ethical relationships and that morality is rooted in the collective life. They see the fundamental nature of a relational ethic lying in ethical commitment and responsible agency. They define the space between moral agents as a relational space for discovering knowledge about others through dialogue and sensitive interaction.

Four themes are identified and developed in the book. *Engagement* is the first, and this requires facing both rational and emotional aspects of others' lives. A layered approach is suggested, encouraging co-existence of subjectivity, objectivity, and interactive engagement in a dialectic that allows strangers to engage in an ethical way.

Mutual respect, the second theme, provides the ethical space to explore with empathy differences between individuals, views, cultures, kinds of knowledge, and systems. It acknowledges the circular and reciprocal nature of giving and receiving.

Embodiment is a term the authors use for the third theme, which focuses on "bringing knowledge back to life" through stories that describe life in an evocative manner. Such narratives enable one to "be with" others in what they call "nonlinear time"—time that is not measured in the duration of interpersonal contact, but rather in the quality of deep and meaningful interaction. We can all think of occasions in our lives when in a "flash" we have "connected" with a person at a crucial moment through a "story," in a way that may not have happened under other circumstances of much longer duration.

The fourth theme, the creation of an ethical *environment*, rejects an individualistic framework as too narrow and calls for solidarity within a web of relations. Provided is a soul-searching example of a wheelchair-bound woman with spina bifida who considers herself normal and is pregnant with a girl-child known to have spina bifida. Here the decision whether to abort such a pregnancy cannot be made merely by the woman as an isolated individual, because of the ramifying ethical and practical implications for her and those with whom her life is emotionally and practically intertwined.

Relationships are described as "processes without end," and relational space is seen to serve as a bridge between micro ethics (interpersonal ethics) and macro ethics (with global implications), by giving due consideration to individuals and community. In a world in which money, power, bureaucratic processes, the law, technology and self-directed action increasingly dominate life, there is a great danger of eroding the generosity, self-effacement, sharing, love, compassion, empathy, and solidarity required to link each of us to many others—within families, small communities, countries, and the world. The capacity to imagine a better future is an integral aspect of macro-ethical relationships.

The authors make it clear that the relational ethics they describe and advocate do not undermine the usefulness of ethical theory, principles, rules, and guidelines. They acknowledge the necessity for acquiring value-free, factual knowledge and applying analytical reasoning. However, they point out that, as the foundational knowledge for relational knowledge is found in understanding the other, it is also necessary to explore the milieu in which ethics is practiced and culturally embedded.

To achieve this, dialogue is vital. Here language becomes critical, and the requirement is for language that is dialogical, collaborative, and interactive rather than defensive, commanding, and impositional. A moral language that is richer than "rights language" is needed, and languages of responsibility (justice) and responsiveness (care) must be included. Power is also an important consideration, and the point is well made that "power over," enabled by technology, needs to be leavened by "power with" that requires mutual respect and "empowerment" through such processes as informed consent.

The state of the world today, threatened by conflict, widening disparities in wealth and health, lack of access to decent living conditions, and inadequate achievement or respect for human rights, calls for new paradigms of thinking and action. Maintaining the status quo or making minor changes are insufficient to reverse current trends. Relationships are important and need to be studied and improved at many levels. While it seems obvious to begin with relationships between individuals, the analysis provided and the methods advocated can be applied to building much needed ethical relationships within and between communities, institutions, nations, and our environment.

Solomon R. Benatar
Bioethics Centre
Department of Medicine
University of Cape Town

Introduction

It all started over lunch. Some years ago the two of us, John Dossetor and Vangie Bergum, decided on lunch at the Faculty Club at the University of Alberta. As we chose our meal from the generous, varied buffet, we looked over the river valley, and talked. We had been puzzling about the notion of autonomy that was so prevalent in the bioethics literature that we used in our classes with graduate students. What is the responsibility, authority, and limit of autonomy? How does our understanding of individual freedom relate to community responsibility? What is the meaning of personhood? How does the belief that all people are morally equal reflect itself in practice? Can ethics really be taught? Can attention to ethical practice enhance the ethical thinking learned from theory?

Since that lunch, we have come to understand that healthcare ethics is not *only* an objective discipline—a theory that accords authority and privilege to the careful and consistent application of definitive principles to action—but is also a *relationship*. In relationships we have the opportunity for dialogue between theorists and practitioners, between rationality and hermeneutic knowledge, and between healthcare professionals and patients, and this relationship becomes the core, the ethical source that guides actions. This book is the result of a research endeavor that arose from the ideas and questions pondered over during that lunch hour. We joined together in planning and conducting what came to be a fascinating, challenging, and fruitful project. We gathered together a wonderful array of professionals and academics to ponder how to think about, and even how, to continue to nurture ethics in our healthcare environments. Our colleagues, members of the Interdisciplinary Research Group, are listed in appendix A. This book is a result of the work of this team, first as members of the Interdisciplinary Research Group, and then as contributors to the ideas and editing of this book. The collaboration among this group has been a defining characteristic of this project. Throughout the text we have referenced the material that comes directly from the transcripts of the various meetings, but the text itself represents the knowledge and experience gained throughout the whole project. In appendix B we identify the dates and time of the meetings of the Interdisciplinary Research Group.

Sandra McKinnon, a member of our research team, suffered through cancer during our research program. Before she died on 9 September 2000, we told her that this text would be dedicated to her. Now, when her colleagues—from the palliative care unit where she was manager—find themselves in situations of conflict or with moral questions they think, "What would Sandy have done? Is this how she would have acted?" Clearly, Sandy's legacy lives on.

The research, funded by the Social Sciences and Humanities Research Council of Canada, was designed to contribute to the development of knowledge and practices in healthcare ethics by deepening our understanding of the nature and importance of relationships between people and of their responsiveness to each other in the context of ethical reflection and decision making. Hours of discussion by the research team, hundreds of pages of transcripts, numerous days of analysis, and various activities by student researchers, led to a variety of outcomes. We wrote and produced a video, accumulated a number of photos and paintings, which were been made into slides for use in presentations, secured additional funding for related research projects, and began work on written texts.

Some ideas that were seeded during the research have developed and flourished through careful tending; others have been taken by the wind to fall in the wild like weeds. At one of our research meetings, a member of the Interdisciplinary Research Group said, "I find these meetings to be very stimulating, and I go away with a bunch of ideas. Sometimes one or two crystallize, and I can reflect on them for a while, write them down, throw them back in the pot, and see what happens. I would like to learn more about ideas like mutual thinking and 'the space between.' I am thinking that maybe nurturing ethics involves nurturing the space between people and nurturing the ability to extend oneself into that space. I love the fertile ground found here—ground where ideas get planted and where time is given to allow us to go away and ruminate and then feed something back in. I don't know where this all will lead. Probably just fodder or grist for the mill."[1]

No *final conclusions* have come out of this research. Rather, the ideas discussed in the project led us to write a text as a way to continue the dynamic conversation that planted the first seeds of this project. The text is written with the intent to explore ways to open up our thinking about ethical commitments in health and healthcare. We may, in the end, see this text and the research project as our way of *nurturing ethics*— nurturing broad discussions of health ethics in order to stimulate others' ideas. These ideas do add fodder or grist to our search for better understanding of our ethical commitments to ourselves, to one another, to the healthcare environment, and to the earth. We may, in the end, see our work as that of nurturing the space that can hold the dialectical tension between principles and care, between scientific and experiential knowledge, between what we should do and what we can do, and, even between what is good and what is not good. A relational space may be a place where there is a flow between rationality and embodiment, between the challenges of the thinking mind and the realities of the feeling body. A relational space is found both between people as well as within each person.

Nurturing a relational ethic does *not* leave behind normative ethical principles, but rather brings mutually enhancing principles together with attitudes and practices of care and respect. The principles are how we attend to the general part that can be abstracted down to the skeleton—the bare bones of how we might characterize ourselves abstractly. Getting to know the bones of the person is like getting to know the basic principles. The principles are always essential as a sort of guarantee that we will attend, at least, to that general part, the objective part of the person. But we suggest that our ethical responsibility and commitment cannot stop there—with principles and generalizations. Rather we propose that through relationship we put flesh on the bones of personhood. To get to know each other in a much richer and more detailed way, we see each person in their fullness and complexities—more than just the bones. Nurturing the space between us shows the respect that is found in getting to know each person. Relationship is the drama of nurturing ethics—a drama that theory can never illustrate. This text is a conversation about how to nurture ethical understanding and ethical action. It is not about normative ethical theory. We propose that without this integral element of relationship there is danger that ethics, itself, falls away by virtue of having nothing to support it.

Nurturing the space between us, *as an ethical task*, is a fascinating thought. In fact, nurturing the relational space has evolved into the central attention of our work. In many professional disciplines we talk about the importance of the professional relationship with the people served, or even between and among professionals themselves. Professions are, in reality, characterized by the commitment to relationship—the therapist-patient relationship, the doctor-patient relationship, the clergy-family relationship, the doctor-nurse relationship, and so on. In this text we want to foster a deeper, more integrated attention to relationships between people—an attention and acknowledgment of the space between people. The space between, then, becomes an entity or thing in itself, not controlled by one person or the other but as a space that holds people in relation—a *third* entity—to which both people contribute. Some have called this space a third space or a *dialogical space*. But, of course, this space cannot be an entity by itself. Like the trunk of a tree, such a space is nothing without roots and branches. A tree trunk, like ethical space, cannot live alone.

We call this space the *relational space* or ethical space, and the ethical themes that we uncovered through our research live within this space—themes of mutual respect, engagement, embodiment, uncertainty and possibility, freedom and choice, and environment. Consider the thematic notion of mutual respect. How might the notion of mutual respect be developed within this relational space? We propose that mutual respect can be expressed only in a space or moment that gives equal attention to the needs, wishes, expertise, or experience of both parties to the relationship. Mutuality, as such, is not something that can be applied by the caregiver to the relationship. Rather, mutuality and mutual respect develop between both parties in the relationship—in that relational space between.

Some might see this ethical approach as too unstructured, lacking the logical control expected from scientific or philosophical rationality. Others may feel that such an approach would lead to relativism—a worry that is found in the idea that anything goes depending on the specific circumstances—that nothing can ever be absolutely right or absolutely wrong. Others, too, might find it too idealistic—not possible in our current fast-paced world of healthcare. We, however, suggest that the commitment to fostering ethical space may be the only way to ethically approach different values, different beliefs, different cultures, difficult kinds of knowledge, different genders, and so on. Relationship, from an ethical point of view is, in fact, held together by respect for difference—and that respect for difference is both rational and a protection from relativism. A focus on relationship holds the tension between particular preferences, feelings, and opinions and the general moral good of humanity, normative guidelines, and community values. *Relationship* and its demands may be the very place where we need to put our attention in this time of moral upheaval, economic disparity, human rights abuses, and fears of evil. A focus on relationship, the spaces between people, between people and agencies, between agencies and government, between nations and cultures, recognizes that there are possibilities for moral development, opportunities for new ways of thinking about responsibilities, and of enhancing the use of technological successes for the good of all people. Within a relational approach we take all differences into the relational space—not holding "us" close and banning "them," not seeing us or this activity as "good" or the other as "bad." Rather, a relational approach desires that together we face the reality of both/and—*both* the rational *and* the emotional, the successes and failures, and the good and the evil that permeates all of us. Relational ethics, then, is the flow that is made possible by a focus on the space between us—a space in which we can nurture ethical discussion and develop ethical thought.

In each of the following chapters, we build a relational ethic based on relational space through contemplation of the themes that were identified in our research.[2] In each chapter we gather concrete examples to consider the identified themes. These examples illustrate the value of narrative as a way to bring the reality of personal human experiences to light. The advantage of story is that the readers can engage with the people and circumstances from their own perspective—can extend the story by relating it to their own life experiences and see the truth in it for themselves. Perhaps studying relationships in one situation tells something about all other relationships. Each experience of relation could be representative or symbolic of the whole. Each experience of being in a relationship can maybe tell us something about the greater relational ethic.

In chapter one, we focus on the research project itself, as we describe gathering in the library where original discussion and thinking occurred. In this library it became clear to us that the relational ethic that we were attempting to discover and articulate for health situations is the same ethic that we hold in the space between us as researchers and research participants, teachers and students, friends and neighbors, and, dare we say, between enemies. The time, intensity, intent, and purpose of the situations may be different, but the themes may be the same. The space between holds the micro to the macro, the individual to the system, and the system to the world. In our library, the location of the research, the ethical consciousness needed to develop the spaces between us were the same *in here* (in the research project) as they are *out there* (in the healthcare system). Readers fascinated by different research approaches used in the human sciences might find this chapter particularly interesting. Readers less interested in the nitty-gritty of research procedures might wish to move directly to chapter two, where we place our relational approach (and place ourselves) within a broad overview of ethical thought.

In chapter two we situate our approach to relational ethics within current ethical thought and practices heuristically, using the insights of American healthcare professionals Edmund Pellegrino and Sally Gadow. We describe how a relational focus is timely, given our current theoretical and scientific emphasis and our current health and world situation. We show how we incorporate philosophical positions with real-life circumstances to find a situation where philosophy and practice function together. We propose the creative use of dialogue to formulate, articulate, and dissolve moral dilemmas that arise in healthcare. We know that there is no aspect of healthcare or research that lies beyond ethical concerns such as those found at the end of life, mid-life or beginning of life, value-based questions of justice in resource distribution, or environmental ethics. We identify fundamental concepts that we come back to throughout the text—being a person, fostering community, and the need for attention to the ethical question in our search for ethical understanding.

In chapter three we begin to explore more deeply the theme of mutual respect. We begin the discussion by gathering around the infant K'aila, through his parents' story of their decision to withhold transplant treatment from him. This story provides a rich opportunity for us to explore the notion of mutual respect. The word *respect*—itself through attention to its etymological Latin root *respectus*, which means to regard, to look back—helps us to develop a more meaningful understanding of the importance of respect. When we add the adjective *mutual* to the notion of respect, this relational ethical theme becomes both more significant and more complex.

Chapter four invites us to gather around Dax, the central person in the well-known story of the severely burned man who wished to be allowed to die. Although since the early 1970s, when Dax's tragic injury took place, society has come to be more respectful of an individual's autonomous wishes, this story helps us to think about how we engage each other in understanding and developing our ethical commitments. In this chapter we question whether engagement between people is possible in the current healthcare environment, which is becoming more and more market driven and more interested in outcomes (ends) than on how to reach the outcomes (process). We suggest that engagement is not only possible, but is ethically necessary.

In chapter five we reflect on the story that a family brought to our research meetings. The family told us about removing a feeding tube from Allison, a young woman who had suffered a tragic car accident. They told us how they came to their final important ethical decision by maintaining a close relation with their daughter and sister. They did not turn away from Allison's life to contemplate ethical theory as they struggled with understanding what was the right thing to do. The family brought life into ethics by showing us how, through living *with* Allison, they came to know what they should do with and for her. In this chapter on living and dying, we explore the integration of the feeling body with the thinking mind. In this chapter we consider the strength and value of broadening the notion of rationality to include knowledge gained from attending to the knowledge of the lived body.

In chapter six we explore the notion of the ethical environment. Again we envision a relational space where we are not caught dualistically, with the care of patients "here" and the healthcare system as environment "out there." Using a now-frequent experience of parents' decision making following prenatal diagnosis, we explore the notion of freedom and choice and suggest that individual freedom be hooked to responsibility to our larger community. The relational space, in actual life, ties the individual to the healthcare system, to the globe, and to the earth. The environment is *us*—not "us" versus "them"—but *us*, all that is *us*. We suggest that with each action, each moment where we decide something on the basis of what we should do rather than what we can do, we create a new environment. Thus changing the environment occurs moment by moment. We propose that the individualistic freedom of liberal philosophy is too narrow an understanding to appreciate the interdependence found through the relational lens.

In chapter seven we contemplate the technological "house" that we live in. We identify a number of factors that have led us to this house: objectification, professional codes, and the marketplace. We consider the implications of living in our technical house and invite a return to relationship. To heed the call to relationship, we realize that we need to "let go of the script" so the relationship can follow its own lead. While we can let go of the script, we know that we cannot abandon it. We suggest that the major themes of the text— mutual respect, engagement, embodiment, and environment— prevent a fall into relativism. As a call, relationship is not seen as a mandate or an absolute requirement, but relationship is a process without end. In this chapter we summarize the themes of the text and invite readers to consider ways to keep the conversation going.

While we have attempted to focus on a specific theme within each chapter, the reader will notice how difficult this is to do, as the themes tend to overlap within and between chapters, just as life encompasses all parts of us, even though at times only one part is foremost. With chapter seven we complete the text and invite readers to use the text to reflect on their own professional and personal relationships.

We end this introduction with the words of a Canadian native Cree leader, George Erasmus, from a newspaper article, "Why Can't We Talk?" He says, "the greatest challenge to the world community in this century is to promote harmonious relations between peoples of disparate origins, histories, languages, and religions."[3] Erasmus believes that we "have the capacity to imagine a better future, and we have the tools at hand to realize it. Let us decide now to pursue our common goals together, to achieve long life, health, and wisdom for all, good relations and peace between peoples, and respect for the Earth that supports us." We offer this text as a contribution to the dialogue—the talking together—that needs to happen in order to move toward lofty goals of good relations and peace between people and the place in which we live.

NOTES

1. Ideas from the transcripts of the Interdisciplinary Research Group and Research Team Discussions are included throughout the text. Citation is given only for direct quotes and only identified by the code number of the meeting as indicated here: Interdisciplinary Research Group #7.

2. See the following where ideas, developed in this text, were first published: Wendy Austin, Vangie Bergum, and John Dossetor, "Relational Ethics," in *Ethics in Nursing: Issues in Advance Practice*, ed. V. Tschudin (Woburn, Mass.: Butterworth-Heinemann, 2003), 45-52; Vangie Bergum, "Discourse: Ethical Challenges of the 21st Century: Attending to Relations," *Canadian Journal of Nursing Research* 34, no. 2 (2002): 9-15. Vangie Bergum, "Relational Ethics for Nursing," in *Toward a Moral Horizon: Nursing Ethics in Leadership and Practice*, ed. J. Storch, P. Rodney, and R. Starzomski (Toronto, Ont.: Pearson Education Canada, 2004), 485-503.

3. George Erasmus, "Why Can't We Talk?" *Toronto Globe and Mail*, 9 March 2002, F6-7.

1

Ethical Relations in Healthcare

INTRODUCTION

We begin with two stories of women with their caregivers. Each story takes us to the heart of this book—ethical relations in healthcare. In both of these stories the patient is dying.

THE FIRST STORY

During the last 18 months of my mother-in-law's life, my wife spent much of her time caring for her. Finally, near the end, we decided to put Alice [the mother-in-law] into the hospital and found a bed on a palliative care ward. Once again my wife was introduced to yet another professional and prepared herself to tell the whole sad story of her mother's illness in all its gory detail as she had been forced to do so many times to so many different caregivers over those 18 months. But this time there was a difference. The healthcare professional who sat down with my wife said, "Tell me about your mother. Don't tell me about her illness. Tell me about her as a person. What kind of a woman was she? What did she do in her life? What were her joys and sorrows?"[1]

THE SECOND STORY

The other day a healthcare professional told my wife, Gwen, that if she had a cardiac arrest, she would not be resuscitated. Gwen asked me, "How can they do that? Yes I have metastatic disease, yes my lungs are bad, and yes I understand I will die, but I want to be resuscitated should I die tonight." You know, my wife has enough to cope with without this. It is as though they keep saying to us, have you figured out yet that Gwen is dying? Well we know, but we are just trying to live our lives and live through this. Sometimes I think they would be happier if we both would just lie down on the bed and die now. But we still have our dog to care for, I still have my job, our life rhythms go on until she dies. And we have to have some hope for the next minute, the next hour. They try to take that away from us because they are afraid we have not understood, and they won't have fulfilled their medical mandate to tell us. But we know. Tell them we know. We still have to live somehow. They make it difficult.[2]

Even in dying, we live every day, each moment.

These stories talk about ethical moments in healthcare practice—ethical moments that can be enlivening or defeating. Little moments (just one conversation) that make a difference in the dying person's life and death. These close-up ethical moments point to the importance of relationships of healthcare professionals and patients with their families. These close-up moments point to the concrete experiences of life's tremors. Relationships, as ethical moments, can be about big decisions such as euthanasia or abortion (governed by principles, virtues, or codes), but they are also about the qualities found in the moments—how we talk with patients, what attitudes we hold, and how to use the power that is present. These moments in practice are always about relationships, as our actions, according to Walter Jeffko, "cannot occur in a vacuum; the self needs an other with which to interact. Action, therefore, is inherently relational."[3] Ethical practice, as presented in this text, explores the nature of relationships within healthcare—relationships among caregivers themselves and with the persons in their care.[4] When we focus on ethical practice (where ethical interaction takes place), relationships become important and significant sources of ethical insight and responsibility.

The relational approach to ethical practice has seen a surge of interest in the 1980s and 1990s—a time when trust and belief in the ability of science, technology, and rationality to answer all our health problems began to wane. Until recently, Western bioethics literature focused on (1) principles and rules, that point to right action; (2) virtues, that point to right character; (3) casuistry, that points to prior cases and situational analysis; and (4) caring, that points to the need for attention to the particularity of persons and the responsibility and compassion of caregivers. Knowledge of ethical theories, principles, traditions, virtues, or care are vital in any approach to healthcare ethics, yet there is a need, in each approach, to more fully explore relationships in which the ethical moment is enacted. When we speak of ethical practice, we consider practice at all levels, at the bedside and in the community, in policy development, in research, and in education. Relational ethics, a complex and comprehensive layer of ethical thought, builds on ethical theories, principles, virtues, and care.[5] This text, and the research on which it is based, responds to questions such as those raised by Robert Veatch: Can one be morally indifferent to relationships as long as principles are applied? Can one be morally indifferent to relationships as long as the virtues of people are defendable?[6]

We propose that some kinds of relationships are better than others for healthcare practice, and, through the insights gained from the Relational Ethics Research Project and current literature, we outline the basic tenets of an ethical relation.[7] Of course, a relational approach to ethics is already practiced in many areas in healthcare, yet there remains a need for a well-developed perspective that gives voice to the significance of ethical relationships and how to improve them. As a practice ethic, a relational ethic looks at the way persons *are* with one another in various roles: as healthcare practitioner, patient, team member, teacher, student, parent, neighbor, as well as friend. Such a focus attends both to who one is, as well as what one is or does, as we live ethical action moment by moment. We invite readers to consider the ethical insights that come from immediate daily practice and the ethical actions generated from relationships between persons, caregivers, and patients, in real-life situations. Often these real situations bring our attention close to the bedside, the reality of acting ethically. We also invite readers to consider how attention to relationship can influence ethical action in locations some distance from the bedside—between healthcare professionals, administrators, policy makers, and so forth.

Based on the premise that positive nurturing relations are fundamental to growth, healing, and health, the Relational Ethics Research Project was conceived. The research was designed to contribute to the development of knowledge and practices in healthcare ethics by increasing understanding of the relationships between people and their responsiveness to each other. The healthcare relation, as a distinctive kind of relation, is ethical as well as clinical, in that an individual (and often others, such as family and friends who are important to that individual) looks to the healthcare practitioner for support in growth, healing, and dying. The reality of attending to the needs of people during experiences of birth and death, health and illness, make the ethical concerns of healthcare relations particularly challenging.

The healthcare system, and those who work in this system, are informed by moral ends[8] and are governed by mission statements and codes of ethics that contain normative declarations that relationships ought to be of a specific kind— a kind that fosters the good of both the individual and society. Indeed, relations between people, all people, hold the possibility for promoting the good, the occasion for human flourishing, where persons have opportunity and freedom to be the best they can be. The word *flourish* brings to mind images of growth, opening, expanding, and thriving—images that need to be examined in their full meaning, as one way to keep humanness alive and well. There is a need to find, indeed to recover, words and images that remind us of the qualitative difference between surviving and living, disease and well-being, or curing and healing. We need to reconsider the prospect of healing even in the face of death. By exploring human flourishing in these broader ways, we see death as a valued part of life itself and not as something to be feared or even perceived as a failure of medicine. Human flourishing (*eudaimonia*) is not just happiness or a feeling of satisfaction (a static state), says Martha Nussbaum, but rather emphasizes activity and actively focuses on living life in its fullness.[9] Actively living life has to do with relationship with the self and with others. We propose that human flourishing, as personal and societal health, can be enhanced through healthy and ethical relationships.

This chapter gives an overview of the research project: its intents and purposes, its beginning, its approach, and methods. Readers not particularly interested in the drama of the research itself can go directly to chapter two, where we situate our approach to health ethics within the current discourse. In chapter three we begin with the theme of mutual respect where the person, as patient or caregiver, is central to the discussion. We now turn to the research project itself, which began by gathering in the library.

RESEARCHING RELATIONAL ETHICS

GATHERING IN THE LIBRARY

It was a Saturday morning in late June. The library at the University of Alberta Ethics Centre filled with people. This library, a small room lined with journals and books, is housed in an old building where one can still open windows. The slowly rotating fan added to the recognition that it was a hot summer weekend day. We began with introductions: mental health nurse, pediatrician, lawyer, midwife, gerontologist, theologian, oncology nurse, anthropologist, physical therapist, philosopher, nephrologist, family doctor, community health nurse, psychologist, administrator—a varied group with different backgrounds but with a mutual curiosity to explore healthcare ethics from the point of view of practice. Not only did these individuals have diverse experiences as practitioners, teachers, and/or researchers, but the group as a whole varied in gender, prestige, power, and ethnic background. In spite of the differences between us, we were largely a group of well-educated, active, healthy, White, middle-class individuals—even though, even here, illnesses experienced by ourselves and others in our families were present in our minds.

We lived in a society where comprehensive, universal, and publicly funded healthcare benefits were available to each of us. In many ways, we were a privileged group. This group, called the Interdisciplinary Research Group (IRG), met regularly for two years to explore healthcare ethics from the perspective of practice. In fact, the group has stayed connected in subsequent years, leading to a number of other projects.[10]

Because the research took place in the library, and not in the clinic or hospital, we discussed healthcare situations by use of videos, photographs and art, and personal and family stories. Concrete examples brought to the IRG discussions included three actual situations: *Dax's Case: Who Should Decide?*[11] a video about a severely burned person who was treated against his will; *A Choice for K'aila: May Parents Refuse a Transplant for their Child?*[12] a video about parents whose infant son risked apprehension by social welfare because the parents would not consent to a liver transplant for him; "Allison's Story," a personal recounting by three family members of one family's decision to remove the feeding tube of a comatose daughter and sister; and a fictitious story about choice following prenatal diagnosis, in the video *Who Should Decide?*[13] Early in our work, however, we discovered that our learning about relationships was actually experienced within our research group itself, where we met the challenges of relationship head-on. All IRG meetings and some research team discussions were audiotaped, transcribed, and analyzed. The meetings of the IRG were engaging, challenging, personal, intense, and, at times, not long enough, as the discussions often continued on into the parking lot. While the library was the focus of regular research discussions during the first years of the project, the IRG continued to meet over the subsequent years. The members were engaged with the project to the end, have read drafts of this text, and inspired its continued development.

PURPOSE OF THE RESEARCH

The overall purpose of the Relational Ethics Research Project was to develop a comprehensive and philosophically grounded relational ethic for healthcare. The objective was to turn thinking about ethics and our ethical commitments to the reality of how and where we experience them—within healthcare practice. The research was designed to contribute to the development of knowledge and practice of healthcare ethics by increasing understanding of the ethical commitments (connections) between people. As we reflect on the nature and role of ethics, specifically healthcare (or biomedical) ethics, from the point of view of actual clinical situations, we begin to see how central relationships are to ethical practice. In this text we also consider the interdependent and complex nature of relationships of people and environment, and consider Kent Peacock's assertion that ethics is not social, political, or rational, but ecological.[14]

The importance of our research is in the development of an ethic that reflects concepts, theory, practice, and, according to Susan Sherwin, in "models of human interaction that parallel the rich complexity of actual human relations and . . . recognize the moral significance of the actual ties that bind people in their various relationships."[15] Theories, principles, and rules are thus placed within the context of culturally, technologically, and socially diverse relationships. Deep respect for each other, both as practitioners and people using a healthcare system, is required by such relationships.[16] The idea of finding a universal solution in ethics is placed in question in order to explore morality as it is acted out through interpersonal activity set in a unique local context.[17] Instead of searching for universal principles for application (which is another task), we, in this research, explore the notion that relationships are the location for ethical action, and thus are the source of ethical questions and concerns as well as ethical understandings.

A relational ethic can also be strategically important for the development of healthcare policies in two main categories: (1) policies influencing the conduct of healthcare professionals and the quality of individual healthcare delivery, and (2) policies determining the allocation of resources for the support of programs. Currently, in the first category, micro-allocative policies remain focused on individuals who are involved in healthcare. These individuals include patients, clients, students, healthcare professionals, and educators who aim to improve quality in healthcare through positive personal and professional relations. When the focus is on a particular patient or professional, attention to the larger community can be lost. This is exemplified by the professionals' focus of attention on the individual patient with little consideration of the needs of the community. In the second category, where macro- and meso-allocative decisions are made, individuals (in their particularity) are usually functionally removed from the discussion. In policy decisions, the individual people affected by policy determinations are not visible to those who establish such decisions. Rather, those directly affected are seen primarily in terms of groups (with individual members treated as identical, equal, autonomous, and statistical) or populations (often, using business terminology, described as customers and/or consumers).

We propose that a relational ethic, as a concrete, action ethic, can begin to bridge the duality of macro- and micro-ethics by envisioning a relational space. In this non-dualistic space, the concerns of the individual as a whole person are considered in macro decision making, and the concerns of the whole community (groups of whole persons) are brought to the awareness of micro decision makers. We begin to ask questions about the traditional separation between the macro- and micro-allocative decisions by pointing to the relationship and interaction between them. Policy makers, administrators, and workers at all levels in a healthcare system need to participate, as partners, in discourse about such relationships so that everyone in the community is valued in equal degree. The urgent problems of our contemporary life (hunger, poverty, population growth, environmental decline, inferior status of women, poor health of children, discrimination, violence, et cetera) will not be well handled without, as Martha Nussbaum put it, "the eye to the good of all human beings, and, indeed, of the entire world."[18] The focus of relational ethics is on people (whole persons) and the quality of the commitments between them. These commitments are experienced in a relational or ethical space, which stimulates a fundamental shift in how to think about health ethics. The shift is from *solving* the ethical problem to *asking* the ethical question. It is a shift from focus on the person as an individual (static, bearer of rights) to the person as an interdependent agent (engaged in activity for one's own flourishing, both autonomous and as part of the world community).

One question, and the most challenging, perhaps, is: What certainty can be expected in the development of ethical knowledge? Our claim is that ethical knowledge cannot be known ahead of time; rather, ethical knowledge must be developed in relationship. This claim challenges a sometimes-held expectation that ethical knowledge can be secured once and for all time, or can be held as "expert" knowledge by a privileged few (bioethicists, clinicians, philosophers, lawyers). Of course, this claim does not mean that we can know nothing ahead of time: we do know ethical theory and principles, clinical expertise, communications skills, and so forth. The post-modern challenge of many truths is not to say that there is no truth, but that what is true can be found within the history and the current configurations through which people live out their lives. In practice, and perhaps especially healthcare practice, ethical action often takes place without anyone being absolutely sure of the right thing to do. As Anita Tarzian notes, we need to embrace such uncertainty rather than resist it, so that ethical moments are not lost in the search for certainty or in the fear of uncertainty.[19] We also need to embrace uncertainty because it is crucial to maintaining a relational openness—when truth becomes revealed in the moment. John Caputo rightly says, "We act not on the basis of unshakable grounds but in order to do what we can, taking what action as seems wise, and *not without misgivings*. We act, but we understand that we are not situated safely above the flux and that we do not have a view of the whole. . . . *We act because something has to be done* [italic added]."[20] In practice, ethical certainty is often unattainable. There is no clear, objective, high mountain vantage point where we can "see the world as from no place within it," nor is there any clear sureness found in the deep valley of subjective experience. Rather, as Raimond Gaita said, ethical clarity has to come "inescapably, dialogically, in the midst. There is no other place from which we can have anything to say, or anything to learn, about the kind of meaning of actions and lives."[21]

The fundamental nature of relational ethics is that ethical commitment, agency, and responsibility for self and to the other arises out of concrete situations that invariably involve relations between two or more people and affect two or more people. Responses to the questions, How should I act? or How should I live my life? or What is the right and good thing for me to do? are discovered within these concrete and practical relationships. A relational approach differs from the currently dominant view that holds that universal ethical principles and rules are the primary source of ethical guidance. A focus on relationship suggests that the source of our ethical commitment is grounded in our everyday relations to each other. This focus on relationship affirms the particular over the universal, with attention to the context in which people live. As Jeffko remarked, "To say that moral value refers to the interrelations-of-ends aspect of action—which is action in its wholeness—means that the field of morality consists of interpersonal action, or the relation among persons. When two or more persons are related, either directly or indirectly, their actions have a moral quality: they are moral-type actions; they are morally right or morally wrong."[22]

Yet a relational ethic does not discard the usefulness of ethical theory, principles, rules, and guidelines. Rather, these analytic approaches are necessary as one kind of the knowledge that is needed, from which relationships between people are initiated and sustained. In fact, there is a need to value many kinds of knowledge (personal, theoretical, scientific, embodied, narrative) in thinking about ethical commitments. These different kinds of knowledge need to be discussed in the same room, on the same table, at the same time, instead of trying to keep them in separate places, safely locked away from making a mess. Again we are reminded that foundational knowledge for a relational ethic is not found in the search for more scientific facts, more technological advancement, or from universal principles. Rather, foundational knowledge for relational ethics is found in a different direction, in relational space—a space where understanding another's situation (individuality, experience, and culture) is given equal measure to knowledge of ethical theory and principles. Relational space includes questioning each other's perspective, challenging ideas, and so forth.[23] We began to see that relational space, or relational ethics, requires dialogue. What is fascinating is that while relational space places emphasis on understanding of the other, it implies (in fact, necessitates) understanding of the self.

This research project showed the need for relational space, a space to reflect on relationships. We might describe a relational approach as attending to the art of ethics, which is tied to attributes of love, compassion, and nurturance—subjective attributes of feeling. It is proper, we submit, to use intimate or "close-up" words such as love or nurturance, because health-care touches personal, complex, and profound joys and sorrows of life as lived. The love we speak of here is not intimate in a personal, self-serving, or sentimental way, rather, relational love, which is made of understanding, is person-directed (to both self and other), deliberate, strong, and intentional. Love and understanding could be seen as the same thing, but it might be best to use words other than "love" in speaking about relations between people in healthcare situations. Yet, relational understanding, as it is used in this text, includes the deep care and concern reflected in the word love.

Ethical questions can be approached by exploring the experience of the relationship itself and the obligation that is brought to the practitioners by people asking for care. Particular involvement, commitment, and responsibility in health-care has not necessarily been chosen by healthcare professionals, but is accepted (inherited) as part of the role taken by healthcare practitioners. By the very act of entering into a relationship with a patient who seeks healing, practitioners make an "act of profession,"[24] as Edmund Pellegrino and David Thomasma noted, which is a declaration that they, as health-care professionals, will provide care for those who come to them for treatment. In the wearing of the white coat, the white or pink uniform, or hanging the stethoscope around the neck, the practitioner personifies the special knowledge and skills needed to assist the patient. Although doctors, nurses, and other health professionals may forget that they embody relational understanding in taking on the professional mantle, they strive to relieve the suffering and pain of the people in their care. Yet, they know that they are not above the flux (that is, they do not have the whole picture), but are alongside (side-by-side with) patients, and, in recognizing a patient's suffering, can again recognize their own.

COMING TO THE RESEARCH QUESTION

At first glance, it may seem that a relational perspective is an insecure foundation for morality, as we have come to put deep-seated faith in the certainty available from outside scientific, technological, and philosophical rationality. Generally, as a society, we have come to believe that if we develop more objective, factual, value-free knowledge through scientific research and analytical reasoning, we will, in the end, be able to come to certainty and truth and even be able to control life. In such a world there would be no unhappy surprises, no disease that cannot be cured, no behavior that cannot be predicted, and no ethical problem that cannot be conclusively solved. Within this progressive perspective, which many people are now beginning to doubt, we believe that developing more scientific, abstract, and generalizable ethical knowledge will give us truth and certainty. At first glance, given such a belief in the power of science and rationality, depending on a relational approach may be seen as uncertain and unreliable, indeed, too personal, too subjective, or even too emotional. Yet, as we take a second glance toward understanding and building relationships with each other, we might find the relational impulse as a moral foundation is stronger than first thought, and as Zygnunt Bauman asserts, it may be all we have.[25] "Moral conduct cannot be guaranteed; not by better designed contexts for human action, nor by better formed motives of human action. We need to learn to live without such guarantees."[26] We need to learn that clarity and choices come from a different place, a relational space held by both professional and patient, a relational space that is informed by theory, professional clinical competence, and personal experience and knowledge.

Philosophers who have discussed the significance of relationship in ethics suggest various relationships as exemplary of a relational ethic: I-Thou,[27] friendship,[28] the face-to-face,[29] the caress,[30] maternal-child,[31] parenting,[32] and so on. Adriaan Peperzak, in a book called *Before Ethics*, in pointing to relations with wanderers and strangers, suggests that the simple "hello" is enough to initiate a morally important event.[33] Brenda Cameron, too, shows how the question, "How are you?" has moral significance.[34] She suggests, "When a nurse turns a 'How are you?' into an ultimate gesture of being present for someone, she lives the essence of caring for someone."[35] With patients who have difficulty communicating in response to questions such as "How are you?" or "What is it like?" Oliver Sacks says that the physician must become "a fellow traveller, a fellow explorer, continually moving with his patients, discovering with them the vivid, exact, and figurative language which will reach out towards the incommunicable. Together they must create languages which bridge the gulf between the physician and patient, the gulf which separates one man [person] from another."[36]

It was the mothering relationship that triggered the questioning of a relational ethic in this research study. From her research on mothering, Vangie Bergum proposed that mothering is an important relation in which one (the mother) is, in a moral way, claimed by another (the child) and is the foundational experience of moral connection and commitment.[37] The mother-child relationship is the first opportunity of connection and love that everyone experiences: we are carried in our mother's body (where two bodies are one and one body is two) and are tied to our mothers (even if mothers die or abandon their children). The mother's body creates (by opening) a space for the child and the child creates (by pushing out) the space in the mother—a physical and moral space. The navel is a vivid reminder of this primordial and everlasting connection between people, and, like the first story at the beginning of this chapter, we understand the ethical importance of attending to a mother's dying.[38] The daughter knows how important it is to attend to this woman who gave her life. In the book, *The Worth of a Child*, Thomas Murray asks us to consider parenting commitments to the child when doing ethics.[39] Parenting (relational) commitments need consideration in ethics, along with historical and social contexts, current facts, multiple values, emotional intuitions, as well as received philosophical theories.

Of course all people, all children, do not have healthy beginnings, either in connection to their mothers during pregnancy, or in relations with mothers and fathers as children, yet these early experiences have a crucial impact. Perhaps the importance of these early relations is best recognized when they are missing—the obvious wrong when a mother hurts or neglects her child (even prenatally) or the long-lasting effect on life for those children who are not parented well. In recognizing the importance of these early relationships, we must not mix these significant relational facts with expectations that women and mothers are the primary or natural caretakers of society's children, the ill, the aged, and the disabled. Expectations that women, because of supposedly innate capabilities, should provide the primary caregiving roles may keep them in a subordinated and oppressed place in society.[40] Rather, it is important to recognize what is learned (morally and socially) by society from experiences of pregnancy and mothering, where one turns toward the other—for one to be *with* and *for* the other.[41] The pregnant body and the breast feeding of the infant are images that signal important ways of thinking about relationships as these images show acceptance of difference: the pregnant woman carries within her body another being who may be different from her in sex, race, or ability, and mothers nourish their children to grow to be very different from themselves.[42] Here, space is created for the other. Attention to metaphors that emphasize connections and acceptance, in contrast to traditional metaphors that hold images of power or competition, clarify the need to focus on relationships and a relational ethic. The use of metaphors, for example metaphors of mothering, can only be important for ethics if they bring us back to concrete experience. We need to consider how images of nurturing people who are different than ourselves can help us in our practice.

Although it is important not to place too much attention on where ethical relationships begin, it may be possible to learn lessons from such important relationships. Mothering and parenting, as our primary experiences of relational engagement, are important and dependable precisely because they are personal, because they touch the center of our being and focus on the needs of the mother and father as well as the child. People caught by the powerfulness of the relational claim of others can understand a new father's statement, "I used to be a normal egocentric down-to-earth guy. Now . . . I am less certain of the order of things, less certain that the world revolves around my concerns. What really matters are things I only play a small part in. I have accepted that I'm not the center of things, even within my own world. I know my place."[43] We accept the other's (the child's) claim on us, and this acceptance moves us from a self-centered vision of the world to turn toward the other. It also moves us toward ourselves with these questions: Who are we? How do we want to live?

Not everyone is a mother or a father. Yet everyone is or needs to be mothered—by their birth mother, by their adoptive mother, or by someone else. Every child needs to be mothered; every person needs to be nurtured. Everyone needs support, connection, and engagement with and from others. Luce Irigaray speaks of the erotic relationship in terms of the lover and the beloved that points to the need of people for close, intimate, and supportive relations. She says, "No nourishment can compensate for the grace or work of touching. Touch makes it possible to wait, to gather strength, so that the other will return to caress and reshape, from within and from without, a flesh that is given back to itself in the gesture of love."[44] The experience of mothering, parenting, friendship, or, indeed, being a lover, reminds us that, as Walter Jeffko said, "the unit of personal existence is not I in isolation, but You and I as inherently related to each other."[45] Autonomy, as a rightful individuality, is not lost in this inherent connection, yet the recognition of connection between one another is given full attention.

In our research project, we began by describing relational ethics as an ethic of nurturance, as a way of characterizing the kind of healthcare relationship we are attempting to understand. Nurturance is a concept that conveys that one sustains another through respect and consideration for the other's need or perception of need.[46] The other must at least be aware of a need and also must consent to being helped to meet that need.

One element of nurturance is consent or assent. Yet in a relational ethic, consent is mutual. Consent of the practitioner is
an important element: a professed desire to be committed, to
enter a relationship with the people who come for care and
treatment.

Several overlapping notions need to be acknowledged in
a relational ethic: the nurturing of another person, the nurturing of self, and the nurturing of the relationship. When one
nurtures a relationship, one is not dealing with an "it," but
with a person, a *thou,* through our shared humanness.[47] The
human mutuality of two (or more) persons is what is being
nurtured, and not the communication process itself. While it
may be thought that nurturing of another person is different
from nurturing the relationship, it could be that they are really the same. It may be that through nurturing the relationship, both self and other are nurtured.

To nurture means to give something, something of oneself, not of goods derived from elsewhere or produced from
elsewhere, but something integral to oneself, that is given as a
means of nurturing the other person's need. What is one trying to give? Is it one's professional expertise? Yes, but is that
enough? Is it one's knowledge of the way of the world? Yes,
but what is the particular value in that? Is it to enable the
other to find their own inner strength? Yes, maybe, but this
discussion only substitutes one abstract notion for another
and makes no progress. What then? Perhaps it is giving a part
of one's self—one's humanity—through showing of respect
and willingness to meet another's need.[48] We see then that a
relational view does not pretend that one's professional or
technical expertise is the only need.

What does it mean to say that one gives or shares one's
humanity? Can it ever be defined? One's humanity is the characteristic that makes us different, as a species, from the rest of
the animal kingdom. As humans, we are aware of being persons who are conscious, cognitive, and caring, but we are also
selfish, self-centered, and self-promoting. Our conscious cognition tells us that we have a conflict inside us between wanting to look after ourselves (egoism) and wanting to look after
others (altruism). Another way to reframe this dissonance is
to capture the experience of connection or interdependence

within a network of relationships created and sustained by attention and response. Relational ethics, as a focus on connections among persons, offers a different way of viewing these relations, a way that moves to melding egoism and altruism that is more truly representative of the reality of ethical life. Can one not be for the self and for the other at the same time? Here, the *and* becomes significant—not just the self or just the other. The respected teacher, Ted Aoki, in challenging our individualistic thinking that the self is constituted by alienating the other, points to a saying by Roshin, a Taoist teacher, who says, "Humanity's greatest delusion is that I am here and you are there."[49] Further discussion of the notion of personal relation as "self" and "other" will occur throughout this text.

METHODOLOGY AND PROCEDURES

Philosophical research traditions of phenomenology and hermeneutics are especially useful in exploring ethical relations in healthcare practice because they attend to thoughts, feelings, and behaviors within a shared experience rather than viewed from outside.[50] The research methods that arise from such traditions provide insights that, as Max van Manen notes, "speak not only to our intellectual competence but to our practical intuitive abilities."[51] Scholars in education,[52] healthcare,[53] and other disciplines[54] have developed human science research approaches based on the ideas and scholarship of philosophers such as Edmund Husserl, Martin Heidegger, Maurice Merleau-Ponty, and Hans-George Gadamer.[55] These research approaches are useful in exploring "human situatedness" as a way to understand human life. We chose a human science method for our research in ethics in order to place our questions at the immediate locality of daily life.

As we looked at the particular experience in which ethical moments were enacted, we realized that we were also taking part in shaping and creating the world of ethics. This understanding reflects van Manen's statement that "the world is given *to* us and actively constituted *by* us: reflecting on it phenomenologically, we may be presented with possibilities of individual and collective self-understanding and thoughtful praxis."[56] Attention directed to everyday life, to the living experience of ethical decision making in everyday healthcare practice, helped us to uncover tangible relations. We attended to the words used, the values (both medical and personal) that guided discussion, the patterns that become etched in practices, and the expectations (of both practitioners and persons in their care) that were part of decision making. The following procedures were followed:

- The Interdisciplinary Research Group (IRG) of scholars and professionals met throughout the project, with five or six three-hour meetings each year throughout the first years. Two retreats brought this group together in subsequent years.
- Scenarios were prepared for the meetings of the IRG.
- The meetings of the IRG lasted three to four hours each, were audiotaped, and transcribed as research data.
- The principle and co-investigators and collaborators, along with student assistants, analyzed the research data, identified themes, and prepared summary texts. Some of these meetings were also audiotaped.
- The IRG discussed the identified themes and summary texts for further clarification. IRG members were invited to review texts prepared for publication.

These procedures were reviewed and given the necessary approval by the University of Alberta Research Ethics Committee. The necessary safeguards were set in place regarding protection of confidentiality of persons who were part of the research and for the safekeeping of research data. Consent forms were prepared and used when personal stories of patients and their families were discussed in the research group. The research team agreed on commitments and responsibilities for publishing the outcomes of the research.

As relationships are the most elusive of all realities, yet are seen by many people as the most important and complex element in their lives,[57] we decided to use an interpretive approach. We needed to think of questions that pointed not only to the longevity of relationships, but also to their breadth, and depth. Human life and relationships cannot be explored with attention only to simple chronology, for, as Ken Wilber says, "surfaces can be seen, but depth must be interpreted."[58] So the questions we asked in our analysis included: What is being said? What is meant here? What is another way to look at this issue? What has been missed or overlooked? What else could be said? What about the silences?

A research study that begins with healthcare practice must, we assert, be interdisciplinary, as it purports to study the complexity of issues that cross roles and boundaries of healthcare professionals and related disciplines in the humanities, as well as cultural, racial, and gender differences. Within interdisciplinary work, we needed to recognize the issue of power: How does one avoid any one discipline dominating the conversation? How can one remain aware of the potential that one kind of discipline, gender, ability, or scholarship may privilege the questions being asked and answered? The place of power in relational space will be explored later in the text. Within interdisciplinary work, it is also necessary to respect all points of view as valid moral choices. In our research project described here, we strove for a partnership and a collaborative climate so that knowledge and understanding could be generated that reflected the multi-disciplinary points of view.

Collaboration and discourse are important ways in moving toward resolution of conflict or confusion, but consensus is not always possible. We used a research approach that would increase dialogue and acceptance of difference as an alternative to valuing one dominant approach. By using a research method based on collaborative dialogue between healthcare professionals and scholars from different disciplines, the notions of democracy and respect for difference are constantly in the foreground. In such an approach, keeping the conversation open and alive may have been one of our greatest challenges. In this research approach, ethical action is intrinsic to the research process.

The IRG was able to work collaboratively. This group represented an array of scholars including practicing professionals (clinicians, researchers), graduate and undergraduate students, and consultants. The research group developed into a community where diverse opinions, rationality, and emotions could be expressed. Willingness to consider differing points of view gradually occurred as the ethos of the group became one of trust and respect. Ideas were not only shared but were challenged. It was important that all voices were heard and that disagreement and divergence in thought and action were accepted as valid. Here is an example of the kind of discussion that occurred about the process of the IRG meetings.[59]

> *We may not agree readily. As we get to know each other and have a little more trust we may be able to say some of the things that are a bit more controversial. . . . The fact that I may disagree with someone doesn't mean that I don't trust them. . . . You almost have to have trust to disagree. . . . That's right, so I think the important thing is that we be open to criticism. That doesn't necessarily mean that I have to agree with everything you say. . . . But I hear you saying, too, that we need to keep open about our sureness—criticizing ourselves in a sense. Is that what you're saying?*

We also discussed the diversity of our group and what diversity means to the research.

> *Your preference would be to seek more diversity in the group. Is that the point?. . . . Yes, diversity of world-view, rather than diversity of discipline, which we have. . . . And, are you saying that if we come to agreement very quickly on an issue, that maybe we ought to stop and say, why are we agreeing so quickly on this?. . . . Are there some other views that maybe aren't represented around the table? To question some of our agreement if we come to it easily because, looking around the table, it looks like maybe we are not as varied as we might be.*

Given the diversity and long-term time frame of the involvement of the research team, issues of power, gender, rationality, emotion, and professional hierarchy were present, some more explicitly than others. It became apparent as the process unfolded that the issues we were discussing—ethical actions in healthcare practice—were present in the conduct of the research project itself. The way we listened, how we respected each other, accepted or rejected differing points of view, and how we acted toward each other were exactly the characteristics of the relationships we were studying. We were also aware that, as an advantaged group, we might unintentionally miss attending to the marginalized people and perspectives in our community: the poor, the sick, and the suffering. Even within the research team, we might miss the contribution of the less articulate, or the less philosophically or analytically expert within our group.

The analysis was a lengthy, communal (and often difficult) process. The investigators and research assistants (primarily senior graduate students) read the transcripts of each meeting of the IRG, and together began, through broadly flowing and often lively discussion, to analyze these meetings for relational themes. The process was one of puzzlement, sharing, reflecting, at times consensus, at times disagreement. We were striving to find themes that would illuminate, to capture a sense of what was discussed, and to provide a way to logically and evocatively describe the findings of our research. Some of the subthemes were positive aspects of the theme, and others were negative. For example, one major theme is the notion of *engagement* or *engaged interaction* (see chapter four). One of the positive subthemes of engagement is its mutual nature, while negative subthemes are abandonment and rejection of relationship. The transcripts, reproductions of verbal dialogue, while rich in images, ideas, and concepts, do not completely demonstrate the wide-ranging, embodied discussions that were triggered by this process. Videotaping the sessions might have been helpful in picking up the body language and nuances lost on the audiorecording.

Interpretive analysis is a creative activity, striving for depth of understanding through a circular investigation of situations, exploring both the subjective and the objective aspects. This "movement of understanding is constantly from the whole to the part and back to the whole. Our task is to extend in concentric circles the unity of the understood meaning. . . . Full understanding can take place only within this objective and subjective whole."[60] But even here, we do not lose the distinctions of different kinds of knowledge (experiential as well as normative). Rather, we feel the tension and flow between leaves us to find a new response, a new question. Describing and understanding our ethical commitments from practice demands that we consider all aspects of practice: the place and time, the recipients of care and their backgrounds, the practitioners and their skills, and the circumstances of their meeting together. When we discussed each scenario as presented in a video or narrative, we needed to ask ourselves: How does hearing or seeing only part of the story (on a video, that is already an interpretation) limit our understanding? We had to think about how we would act in the same situation: Could we ever make that situation "ours"? What threads of someone's story resonated with our values? What threads were dissonant? What was our shared humanity?

The desire is to understand the complexity, rather than to make the complex superficial or simple. Understanding complexity recognizes that, as Robert Burch says, "the adequacy of our understanding depending on the adequacy of our questions, and the adequacy of our questions depending on the adequacy of our understanding."[61] Activities that assisted in this circular interpretive activity included reading the text (interviews, group meetings), looking for common themes, asking questions of the text, exploring the language used (colloquialisms, meanings of words, the history, circumstances, culture from which people speak, et cetera), and asking questions from our own practice and experience. Often, in research using an interpretive approach, the writing is done in the first person to show recognition that the researchers "influence, exercise choices, and make decisions about the directions of the research and the conclusions they draw."[62] We have chosen to use the first person in this text (the "we"), to indicate our intent to be fully honest about choices and decisions of the research group.

Although interpretive methods use interviews or group discussions that reflect personal experiences, the interest of our research was not in the individual experience, *per se*, but how personal, subjective experiences spoke to the question of our research. When using examples from healthcare, and when asking practitioners and the persons receiving healthcare to describe their experience, the intent was not to focus on the subjective personal experience, but rather to discover how the particular experience enlarged understanding of ethical relationships. To take another research example: when interviewing women on their personal experience of becoming mothers, the interest is not only, or even primarily, in each woman's subjective experience, but, rather, on how her experience informs the research questions: What is the experience of mothering? How does exploring the experience of mothering point to the nature of the mothering relation?

OUTCOMES

Through the identification of themes, we began to articulate the nature of the ethical relation between healthcare practitioners and persons receiving care. Analyses, in the forms of themes and summaries of the discussion, were taken back to the IRG for further discussion. These themes—engaged interaction, mutual respect, embodiment (embodied knowledge), uncertainty or possibility, freedom and choice, and environment—are the focus of the chapters that follow. Development of the themes, as a means to point to different aspects of healthcare relationship, makes the intangible more tangible. Yet sometimes academic texts are not the best way to describe the experience of relational ethics, so we began to explore other approaches: personal stories, narrative, images (photographs and art), and drama. Personal stories[63] were read and discussed, art and photographs were accumulated,[64] and possibilities of creating a drama began to surface.[65] Visual and literary approaches teach us about ourselves and show us the work we do. They sharpen visual senses, generate new insights and understandings, create interpretive understandings, and promote ethical awareness.[66] In consideration of ethical commitments and decisions, we began to recognize that both the heart and mind must be stimulated, as neither emotion nor rationality alone is adequate.

Interpretive research in ethics does not lead to a theory that can be used to explain or, indeed, to "control" ethical decisions; rather this kind of research invites reflection and theorizing on plausible ethical insights brought from the world of practice. As such, the interpretive methods we used for this research did not result in a decision-making model, nor did they lead to easier answers, but these methods did assist in formulating the ethical questions that needed reflection. The research approach encouraged an attitude of deep respect for the ethical practice of human relations that lead to human flourishing. The practice of healthcare ethics, with its attention to experiences of birth and death, wellness and illness, suffering and compassion, offers opportunities to make a dif-

ference in people's lives at important, and sometimes profound, life junctures. Of course, growth and change occur not
only in people who use the healthcare system, but in those
providing the care as well. Words such as "providers" and
"recipients" already give a place to begin ethical questioning.
What kinds of relationships (power, hierarchical) are indicated
in these words? What would happen if we changed the words?
What would those words be?

Hans-Georg Gadamer reminds us that "the task of making
a moral decision is that of doing the right thing in a particular
situation, is seeing what is right within the situation and lay-
ing hold of it."[67] If ethical care occurs in practice, it cannot be
known ahead of time. Rather, one must attend to the immediacy of the situation and ask: What is going on here? More
often than not, ethical reflection occurs after the fact: Did we
do the right thing? What should we do the next time a similar
situation happens? Of course we prepare ourselves for ethical
practice through discussion of theory and principles as applied to case studies (methods that promote rational, cognitive ways to dialogue about ethics). We also prepare through
art and story (methods that capture intuitive, imaginative, and
aesthetic ways to think about ethics). Situation and context
need careful and critical attention in ethical discussions.

CONCLUSION

Consider again the stories used to begin this chapter.

In the first story, Alice, a mother, was brought to palliative
care, where life and death quiver at this marginal stage of life.
We need to question what knowledge is important for her to
live each moment—until she dies. The nurses and doctors caring for this mother can use objective knowledge without even
talking to her, but they know that they need knowledge about
her as a person—the living "I"—in order to care for her. They
know that they need to find out about her—her joys and sorrows—her, as a person.

Consider, too, the second story. When Gwen's husband
talked about how the caregivers made sure that they knew
that no emergency code would be called if Gwen went into
cardiac failure, he said that this information was protecting

the professionals by filling the mandate to inform patients. It was not caring for Gwen or himself. A week later, Gwen and her husband were talking with her caregiver about their boat. Gwen said, "I want to go sailing one more time and we are thinking of going South next week." The caregiver responded, "South next week, you won't even be alive next week." They were speechless. They couldn't respond. It is difficult for patients and families to deal with comments like that, even if Gwen's own doctor said, "Forget this comment and continue doing and planning what you want to."[68]

The ethical moment experienced by Gwen and her husband cause us to reflect, to ponder. As we feel the horror of the moment, we may feel the seeping away of our own life energies. We see the result of what can happen when our knowledge (she will never survive CPR), judgment (we know best), and interpreted policy (discussing end-of-life decisions with the patient) can cause human suffering. We can certainly sense the patient's suffering as we experience our own. Moments like these call us to relational ethics. Moments like these call us to consider how our behavior can affect others, and to think again of how to give space and time for ethical relationships. Professionals and patients develop relationships over the course (both long or short) of their time together. These relationships can be life enhancing (even in the face of death) and ethical, or they can be life destroying and unethical. Although it is doubtful that Gwen did sail again, her wishing, planning, and sharing these plans with her caregivers showed her desire to *live life fully* right to the end of her life. She wanted to feel the wind in her hair, the water spray on her face, the lure of the open, rolling seas propelling her forward. As she panted for breath with profound air hunger, why deny her this vision? Why not be with her in her experience? After all, we have the capacity as humans to both hunger for breath, and hunger for the wind in our face at the same time.

The central questions to be addressed in this text attend to relationships in the healthcare situation. What is needed for relational ethics in healthcare situations? What kind of knowledge is needed? What is needed in society, as well as healthcare systems and agencies, for ethical relationships to flourish? These themes will be considered throughout this book.

We will consider how engagement can occur, how mutual respect is enacted, how to value embodiment in ethical relationships, how to think about freedom from the perspective of responsibility, how uncertainty contributes to good outcomes, and how vulnerability can be understood as a strength.

We began this chapter with stories of two women dying. We will use story—expressions of ethical moments—throughout the text to show the practical importance of relationships between us. Each chapter is designed to stimulate responses from readers (rewrite the text with your own experiences) in order to continue the dialogue by challenging, and, indeed, extending the work begun by the research and the text. If we accept the notions of interconnectedness—persons as connected—and that ethics requires an attitude of living the questions, then we will come to each situation and relation with an openness to dialogue about what should be done. Such a discussion of ethics in healthcare involves a commitment to listening to individual life narratives of peoples' journey through illness, or major life events, like birth and death. It also means building a new narrative with each other about important life issues. We move away from considering ethics as any prepared or received script, since a script does not allow for the narrative knowledge expressed through the particulars of a personal journey through illness. Narrative knowledge is not something that's an *epiphenomenon*. It's not something that hangs at the edge of rational discourse—something that we just do on the side. Narrative knowledge is something that achieves something very powerful and something that is integral to how we need to understand a world. It is something we do as thinking and feeling people—the presence of feeling and thought. It is principled testimony. Knowledge that comes through story is fundamental to understanding how life is lived and ethical healthcare is practiced.

The notion of principled testimony or principled living as essential to ethical decision making places many voices in the foreground, as many as want to be there. Of course, it may be that some voices are healing while others are strident, yet one might want to consider whose voice is being heard, and whose voice is silent, and why.[69] Decisions made from a relational perspective consider the middle ground, that ever-shifting, wonderful, ambiguous place that we approach with humility, knowing that we are limited, and that none of us ever finally will be in possession of the Truth with a capital "T." Decisions made from a relational perspective weave together emotions, culture, language, rationality, and moral impulses, expressed by mutual understanding and concern.

In this text, we describe a relational ethic in substantive, conceptual, and thematic ways that speak to what such an ethic looks like. We also want to engage you, the reader, in the subject of our interest by offering an evocative text that may be characterized by ambiguity and complexity. [You may, at times, be left with the feeling that one cannot do anything with this text.] The intent of this work is not to give a list of findings, but, instead, to offer a text that may do something to us, to encourage us to act more thoughtfully, perhaps in an attitude of continual reflection, and with more questions. Van Manen identifies a thoughtful text as one that reflects on life while reflecting life.[70] Such a text possesses concrete notions that are experientially recognized. It prompts thoughtful reflection, has an intensity that could be lost with paraphrasing, has a tone that speaks to the braiding of the emotional and the rational, and has the possibility of causing an epiphany, that sudden shift in perspective that changes the way one understands something. These are the goals toward which we strive.

NOTES

1. Daryl Pullman, letter to the authors, 24 December 1998.

2. Brenda Cameron, "Understanding Nursing and Its Practices," (PhD dissertation, University of Alberta, 1998), 237.

3. Walter G. Jeffko, *Contemporary Ethical Issues. A Personalistic Perspective* (Amherst, N.Y.: Humanity Books, 1999), 5.

4. Throughout this book, the words "caregiver(s)," "provider(s)," or "practitioner(s)" include all (professionals, nurses, doctors, attendants, clergy, et cetera) who work with persons in their care (recipients, patients, clients, families, consumers, et cetera) in healthcare situations.

5. Sally Gadow, "Relational Narrative: The Postmodern Turn in Nursing Ethics," *Scholarly Inquiry for Nursing Practice: An International Journal* 13, no. 1 (1999): 57-70.

6. Robert Veatch, "The Place of Care in Ethical Theory," *Journal of Medicine and Philosophy* 23, no. 2 (1998): 210-24.

7. There are two distinct but continuous research projects (funded by the Social Sciences and Humanities Research Council of Canada) that influence this text: Phase 1, *Toward an Ethic of Nurturance*, funded from 1993 to 1997, and Phase 2, *Relational Ethics. Foundation for Health Care*, funded from 1997 to 2001. In Phase 1, six relational themes were identified: engaged interaction, mutual respect, embodied knowledge, uncertainty/possibility, freedom and choice, and environment B. In Phase 2, three specific practice situations (genetic counseling, mental health, and relations between healthcare practitioners) are explored to see how the themes take form in these contexts and whether a relational ethic is broadly useful.

8. See note 5 above, p. 57.

9. Martha Nussbaum discusses *eudaimonia* and the urgency of human suffering as the goal of philosophy. "Eudaimonia is often rendered 'happiness'; but this is misleading, since it misses the emphasis on activity, and on the completeness of life . . . and wrongly suggests that what is at issue is a state or feeling of satisfaction." M.C. Nussbaum, *The Therapy of Desire: Theory and Practice in Hellenistic Ethics* (Princeton, N.J.: Princeton University Press, 1994), p. 15.

10. Other projects of the Interdisciplinary Research Group team include "Called to Oppressive Acts: Mental Health Practitioners' Experience of Moral Distress" (principal investigator, Wendy Austin) and "Relational Ethics: Giving and Receiving Bad News Following Prenatal Ultrasound Examination" (principal investigator, Paul Byrne). The Social Sciences and Humanities Research Council of Canada provided funding for both projects.

11. *Dax's Case: Who Should Decide?* VHS (New York: Unicorn Media for Concern for Dying, 1985).

12. *A Choice for K'aila: May Parents Refuse a Transplant for Their Child?* VHS directed by Frances-Mary Morrison, with Peter Downie (Toronto, Ont.: Canadian Broadcasting Corp., 1990).

13. *Who Should Decide?* VHS, Discussions in Bioethics Series (Montreal, P.Q.: Centre for Bioethics Clinical Research Institute Montreal, 1985).

14. Kent A. Peacock, "Symbiosis and the Ecological Role of Philosophy," *Dialogue* 38 (1999): 703; See also J.S. Robert, "The Complexity of Bioethics, the Bioethics of Complexity," *Health Ethics Today* 11 (2000): 2-5.

15. Susan Sherwin, *No Longer Patient: Feminist Ethics and Health Care* (Philadelphia: Temple University Press, 1992), 49.

16. Robin S. Dillon, "Respect and Care: Toward Moral Integration," *Canadian Journal of Philosophy* 22, no. 1 (1992): 105-32.

17. Kim Lutzen, "Nursing Ethics into the Next Millennium. A Context-Sensitive Approach for Nursing Ethics," *Nursing Ethics* 4, no. 3 (1997): 218-26.

18. See note 9 above, p. 507.

19. Anita Tarzian, "Breathing Lessons: An Exploration of Caregiver Experiences with Dying Patients Who Have Air Hunger," (PhD dissertation, University of Maryland, 1998).

20. John D. Caputo, "Disseminating Originary Ethics and the Ethics of Dissemination," in *The Question of the Other: Essays in Contemporary Continental Philosophy*, ed. Arlene B. Dallery and Charles E. Scott (Albany, N.Y.: State University of N.Y. Press, 1989), 59.

21. Raimond Gaita, *Good and Evil: An Absolute Conception* (London: Macmillan Press, 1991), 142.

22. See note 3 above, p. 17.

23. Robert Burt and Dax Cowart, "Confronting Death: Who Chooses, Who Controls? A Dialogue Between Dax Cowart and Robert Burt," *Hastings Center Report* 28, no. 1 (1998): 14-24.

24. Edmund D. Pellegrino and David C. Thomasma, *A Philosophical Basis of Medical Practice: Toward a Philosophy and Ethic of the Healing Professions* (New York: Oxford University Press, 1981), 209.

25. Zygmunt Bauman, *Postmodern Ethics* (Oxford, U.K.: Blackwell, 1993).

26. Ibid., 11.

27. Martin Buber, *Between Man and Man*, trans. Ronald Greger Smith (New York: MacMillan, 1965).

28. See note 3 above; Lorraine Code, *What Can She Know? Feminist Theory and the Construction of Knowledge* (Ithaca, N.Y.: Cornell University Press, 1991).

29. Emmanuel Lévinas, *Totality and Infinity: An Essay on Exteriority*, trans. Alohonso Lingis (Boston: Martinus Nijhoff, 1979).

30. See note 25 above.

31. Virginia Held, *Feminist Morality: Transforming Culture, Society, and Politics* (Chicago: University of Chicago Press, 1993).

32. Hans Jonas, *The Phenomenon of Life: Toward a Philosophical Biology* (New York: Harper & Row, 1966); RichardJ. Bernstein, "Rethinking Responsibility," *Hastings Center Report* 25, no. 7 (1995): 13-20.

33. Adriaan Peperzak, *Before Ethics* (New York: Humanity Books, 1998).

34. Brenda Cameron, "The Nursing, 'How Are You?' " *Phenom-*

enology + Pedagogy 10 (1992): 172-85.

35. Ibid., 184.

36. Oliver Sacks, *Awakenings* (London: Duckworth, 1973; reprint, New York: Harper Perennial, 1990), 225, n. 104.

37. Vangie Bergum, *A Child on Her Mind: The Experience of Becoming a Mother* (Westport, Conn.: Bergin & Garvey, 1997).

38. Brenda Cameron, conversation with authors, Edmonton, Alberta, October 1999.

39. Thomas H. Murray, *The Worth of a Child* (Berkeley: University of California Press, 1996).

40. Rosemarie Tong, "The Ethics of Care: A Feminist Virtue Ethics of Care for Healthcare Practitioners," *Journal of Medicine and Philosophy* 23, no. 2 (1998): 131-52.

41. Bergum, *A Child on Her Mind*, see note 37 above.

42. Mary C. Rawlinson, "The Concept of a Feminist Bioethics," (paper presented at the International Bioethics Conference, San Francisco, Calif., November 1996).

43. Curtis Gillespie, "The Kid: Commentary on CBC Radio Active," Canadian Broadcasting Company, 9 January 1996, quoted in Bergum, *A Child on Her Mind*, see note 37 above, p. 166.

44. Luce Irigaray, *An Ethics of Sexual Difference*, trans. Carolyn Burke and Gillian C. Gill (Ithaca, N.Y.: Cornell University Press, 1993), 187.

45. See note 3 above, p. 3.

46. Sandra McKinnon, "Nurturance: An Exploration of the Concept," (unpublished paper, University of Alberta, Edmonton, Alb., 1993).

47. See note 24 above.

48. Carol Gilligan, *In a Different Voice: Psychological Theory and Women's Development* (Cambridge, Mass.: Harvard University Press, 1982).

49. Ted Aoki, "Interview: Rethinking Curriculum and Pedagogy," *Kappa Delta Pi Record* (Summer 1999): 180-1.

50. Patricia Benner, ed., *Interpretive Phenomenology: Embodiment, Caring and Ethics in Health and Illness* (Thousand Oaks, Calif.: Sage Publications, 1994).

51. Max van Manen, "From Meaning to Method," *Qualitative Health Research* 7, no. 3 (1997): 345-69, 345.

52. David W. Jardine, *Speaking with a Boneless Tongue* (Bragg Creek, Alb.: Makyo Press, 1994); David G. Smith, *Pedagon: Meditations on Pedagogy and Culture* (Bragg Creek, Alb.: Makyo Press, 1994); see note 51 above.

53. See note 50 above; Bergum, *A Child on Her Mind*, see note 37 above; see note 2 above; Susan James, "With Woman: The Nature

of the Midwifery Relation," (PhD dissertation, University of Alberta, Edmonton, Alb., 1997).

54. Otto Bollnow, *Crisis and New Beginnings* (Pittsburgh, Pa.: Duquesne University, 1987); Robert Burch, "Confronting Technophobia: A Topology," *Phenomenology + Pedagogy* 4, no. 2 (1986): 3-21; Richard M. Zaner, *Ethics and the Clinical Encounter* (Englewood Cliffs, N.J.: Prentice Hall, 1988).

55. Edmund Husserl, *Phenomenology and the Crisis of Philosophy*, trans. by Q. Lauer (New York: Harper & Row, 1965); Martin Heidegger, *Being and Time*, trans. by John Macquarrie and Edward Robinson (New York: Harpers and Row, 1962); Maurice Merleau-Ponty, *Phenomenology of Perception*, trans. by Colin Smith (London: Routledge & Kegan Paul, 1962); Hans-Georg Gadamer, *Truth and Method* 2nd rev. ed., trans. by Joel Weinsheimer and Donald G. Marshall (New York: Crossroad, 1989).

56. Max van Manen, *Researching Lived Experience: Human Science for an Action Sensitive Pedagogy* (London, Ont.: Althouse, 1997), xi.

57. David C. Thomasma, "Toward a New Medical Ethics: Implications for Ethics in Nursing," in *Interpretive Phenomenology: Embodiment, Caring and Ethics in Health and Illness*, ed. Patricia Benner (Thousand Oaks, Calif.: Sage, 1994).

58. Ken Wilber, *The Brief History of Everything* (Boston: Shambhala, 1996), 245.

59. Interdisciplinary Research Group #3.

60. Hans-Georg Gadamer, *Truth and Method* (New York: Crossroad, 1982), 259.

61. Robert Burch, "On Phenomenology and Its Practices," *Phenomenology + Pedagogy* 7 (1989): 187-217, 212.

62. Christine Webb, "The Use of the First Person in Academic Writing: Objectivity, Language, and Gatekeeping," *Journal of Advanced Nursing* 17 (1992): 747-52, 751.

63. See Barbara Rosenblum, "Living in an Unstable Body," *Out/Look* 1, no. 1 (1988): 42-51.

64. A collection of slides of photographs and artwork showing various aspects of relationship or lack of relationship were used to stimulate discussion. These included evocative photographs such as an emaciated woman breastfeeding a small malnourished child, contrasted with a piece of artwork depicting a mother breastfeeding a rosy-cheeked robust infant, a patient lying amidst a plethora of tubes and equipment in an intensive care unit, and a nurse kneeling to speak face-to-face with an elderly patient.

65. . . . *And They Wanted a Child,* a video, was developed to show how a relational ethic might play out at an ethic committee

consultation. The storyline is based on an actual situation in which a woman with HIV and her husband, who suffered from a degenerative muscular disease and a low sperm count, sought assistance from a fertility clinic to conceive a child. The video has been used widely for educational purposes.

66. Philip Darbyshire, "Understanding Caring Through Photography," in *Transforming RN Education: Dialogue and Debate*, ed. Nancy L. Diekelmann and Marsha L. Rather (New York.: National League for Nursing Press, 1993).

67. See note 60 above, p. xi.

68. See note 2 above, p. 238.

69. Robert Burt, "The Silent World: Uncertainty and Medical Authority in the World of Jay Katz," *Law, Medicine & Health Care* 16, no. 3-4 (1988): 190-6.

70. See note 51 above.

2

Situating Relational Ethics in Ethical Theory

INTRODUCTION

Problems of an ethical and moral nature in healthcare have, over the years, been tackled by a number of approaches, each with strengths and limitations. Relationship-based ethical approaches are one way in which scholars (philosophers and healthcare practitioners) have responded to the growing concern that individual rights (liberal-ism), principles and rules (principle-ism), consequences and utility (utilitarian-ism), and impartiality, universality, and rationality (objective-ism) have dominated ethical discourse, leaving out the moral wisdom of prophetic, narrative, and public policy elements.[1] A number of theoretical approaches, such as a communitarian focus,[2] virtue ethics,[3] feminist ethics,[4] an ethics of care,[5] and the resurgence of case-based ethics (casuistry),[6] attempt to widen the thinking. There is concern that all approaches to ethics be well-grounded theoretically and practically and not based on emotion and personal preference nor on the characteristics of the situation without drawing on theoretical and philosophical knowledge.[7] Philosophers such as Raanon Gillon are concerned that any approaches to ethical thought and action "unsupported by a framework for discursive reasoning"[8] will be open to manipulation and abuse. The fear of ethical relativism, be it cultural relativism or situational ethics, is pervasive.[9] The fear is that without a firm theoretical foundation we may fall into moral chaos.

One response that is used to deal with concerns about recent approaches to ethics in healthcare is to develop an even more rigorous foundation of philosophical reasoning. In this direction, the focus of attention is on the nature of ethics through the analysis of the language, concepts, and methods of reasoning in ethics, the study of moral epistemology, and the development of the logic and patterns of moral reasoning and justification.[10] Another response, the one we chose, is to explore and describe ethics from a practical foundation, in which ethical action is experientially and culturally embedded within healthcare practice. It is in this direction that relationships come into focus. Both approaches have validity and are necessary in the continuing development of ethical practice in healthcare.

Contemporary ethical thinking owes much to the moral theories of Kant, Rawls, Mills, and others that led to the development of the bioethical principles of beneficence, nonmaleficence, autonomy, and justice, which are often used in ethical decision making.[11] These theories, often referred to as *theories of justice*, exemplified by principles and rules and by contract relations between equal partners, are based on notions of separateness (individualism, autonomy) and the concern for equality and fairness. The principles of beneficence (do good for the other) and nonmaleficence (do no harm) govern these relations.

Recently, however, there has been recognition of the limitations of a theoretical approach that has been developed from philosophy alone. These concerns question whether normative theory alone is a useful guide for healthcare practitioners, because it lacks sufficient emphasis on the care and respect that are especially needed in chronic and long-term illnesses, and because all relationships are not equal. The four principles, sometimes referred to as the "Georgetown mantra," which Baruch Brody refers to as "middle-level" principles, do not hold a completely unifying approach to ethical deliberation.[12] From the research in relational ethics, we, with other scholars, question the centrality of justice, with its focus on rights, as the *first* virtue of social institutions such as healthcare.[13]

In the early 1980s, Carol Gilligan[14] (among others)[15] challenged the emphasis on legalistic theories of justice in favor of an emphasis on theories of moral development based on connection and care. What is needed is neither justice nor care, says Gilligan, but an ethic that is "fundamentally dialectical in the sense of containing an ongoing tension between justice and care . . . aspiring always to the ideal of a world more caring and more just."[16] Scholars call for an ethical theory and approach based on respect for the interconnection between humans, as well as respect for autonomy.[17] The goal is to achieve a satisfying community with others, as well as to foster personal autonomy and equality of power with others.[18] There is a need to "shake the pillars" of value judgments and absolutes of the past and look for new values and attitudes.[19]

The justice tradition in ethics, which focuses on individual rights, autonomous choice, and contractual relationships, complements the science tradition, as it has come to be construed in recent decades, with its emphasis on objectivity and the search for abstract theory. Robert Burt goes even further to suggest that the scientific approach, with its abstraction, fragmentation, and objectivity, is the forerunner of the emphasis on separateness between people and their world. "The success of scientific medicine during the past half century has prompted physicians to place intense normative value on conceiving themselves as rigidly separate from their external environment, including their patients. This separate, rationally manipulating self-depiction among physicians finds its precise counterpart in the notion that patients should be viewed as separate, rationally manipulating individuals."[20] This extreme abstraction, the disconnection of individuals from one another and from society, is a development of modern society, where ethical language is a language of rights.[21] While emphasis on rights is fundamentally important, it is now timely to explore some of the limitations that have come with rights language and look for a "richer moral vocabulary and vision—not only in private life, but also in public life,"[22] as stated by Gilbert Meilaender. A language that is morally richer would assist in understanding the meaning and significance of a person's death, in discerning the best interests of others (with others), or verbalizing the complex ways that people are harmed or wronged. A richer language calls for responsibility and responsiveness—a language that remembers that moral responsibility, itself, is *the* precious human right—as Zygmunt Bauman says.[23] Within a relational focus there is interest in providing another language, a language that speaks to relation as well as rights, to speak about ethical commitments.[24]

The care tradition in ethics, focusing on the need to take seriously interconnectedness and relationship, is more in concert with ambiguous and idiosyncratic events of actual life experience. Sally Gadow, however, questions accepting *any* ideology (whether it is justice or care), for ideology is theoretical, abstract, values the "general" over the "particular," and could lead to coercion.[25] The opposite of ideology, says Gadow, is relationship. Relationship calls attention to embodied empathic relations that can only be experienced *between* people. Of course, power dynamics exist in relationships, and especially in healthcare relationships, related to two primary issues: (1) the value placed on scientific and medical knowledge and expertise; and (2) the vulnerability and dependency experienced by the ill, and the poor, and/or those who are marginalized by language, culture, race, gender, and so forth. Health decisions are always invested with some kind of power, and this power needs attention and analysis. In chapter three, there will be more discussion of the importance of power to developing ethical relations.

An ethic for healthcare that holds a strong version of both justice and care is, we suggest, one that is grounded in our relational commitment to each other. Within this relational focus comes the exploration of how one person (practitioner, nurse, midwife, doctor, personal care attendant) responds to the obligation brought about by another person (patient, birthing woman, client, baby) and vice versa. A relational ethic acknowledges and extends recognition of the autonomous nature of individual life by developing the notion of *fostering autonomy*, which is founded in the recognition of our mutuality and communal nature of living and making decisions together.[26] As Virginia Held noted, "We should care for one another as persons in need of a habitable environment, with a sufficient absence of violence, and with sufficient provision of care for human life to flourish."[27]

In this chapter, we focus attention on the question, *Where are we?* within the context of the development of ethical theory in Western thought. We explore the connection of relational ethics to traditional ethical theories in both *linear* and *layered* ways. We aim to show that relational ethics is not in opposition to current dominant theories, but a progressive development that reflects where we are at this time in our history, and focuses on issues to which we need to attend. The linear approach takes Edmund Pellegrino's paper, "The Metamorphosis of Medical Ethics,"[28] as a structural source, whereas the layered view builds on the work of Sally Gadow, particularly her paper, "Relational Narrative: The Postmodern Turn in Nursing Ethics."[29] Each of these scholars (a physician and a nurse with a long history of scholarship in healthcare ethics) has a unique perspective that speaks from a disciplinary view. It is timely that scholarly work from both medicine and nursing (as well as other disciplines) is used, given our commitment to interdisciplinary research and discussion of healthcare ethics and the realities of practice, where healthcare professionals must *together* grapple with ethical responsibilities. We, as authors, have learned through our research and through practice that ethical and healing care are best achieved by collaboration between the person who seeks assistance and the healthcare team, and within the healthcare team itself.

As we turn our attention to where we are in bioethics, it is important to ground the "we" in some way. The authors of this text speak from a North American perspective. We seek to give substance to our words through the examples we choose—the Canadian and American history and world view— in the last 50 years. As we speak from this narrow experience, we recognize that it is not the whole picture of ethical thought. Other world-views are equally as valuable, and we begin from this perspective knowing that it is not the whole view. It is our intent to situate ourselves this way in order to continue the conversation that has begun by so many others.

WHERE ARE WE IN BIOETHICS?

As we begin this brief history of bioethics, let us gather around Erika. Erika Nordby captured world news with her dramatic return to life and health from the actual brink of death.[30]

GATHERING AROUND ERIKA
      Erika was 13 months old, living in Edmonton, Alberta, when she somehow managed to push open an outside door of the house and wander out into the neighbor's yard. It was the middle of the night. It was -25 degrees Celsius. She was wearing only a diaper. Her distraught mother found her face down in the snow with her eyes frozen shut, her fingers and toes frozen together. She was not breathing and her heart was still. Erika's frantic mother called 911. The paramedics responded immediately and rushed her to the local hospital emergency ward, where skilled doctors and nurses provided immediate and up-to-date technical and compassionate care. A hovering community waited for news. The child recovered—was brought back to life, it seems. There was no ethical dilemma felt in the immediate care given. Everyone did what was necessary to save the life of Erika. Her mother and all those working in the healthcare system acted from a place of common goals and beliefs. There was no need for deliberation or reflection. Everyone acted immediately.

      The story would have been different if the child's life had been left in a precarious state, not quite living and not quite dying. The professionals and family, together, would have had to make decisions about her ongoing care. The family and healthcare professionals would have needed to deliberate on what course of action was appropriate. They would have looked to the ethical principles to think through the issues. They would have searched for guidance from diverse experts in their deliberations. The parents, the professionals, and even the community would have struggled together to know what to do.
      The story would have been different if the healthcare environment had not been in place: with no 911 at one's fingertips, no ambulance at the ready, no emergency and pediatric intensive care units, no skilled doctors and nurses available, and costs not covered by universal healthcare. The story would

have been different if the hospital refused to treat the child because of an inability to pay, or if Erika had no mother to miss her, search for her, and get her to the hospital. The story would have been different if racial tensions limited care for certain children—children of the wrong color or children who spoke the wrong language.

While the Western world buzzed with the miraculous news of the recovery of this one small child, we know that in many parts of the world children die due to the lack of healthcare resources. Children also die because of impersonal acts of hostility and war, or alone in orphanages for want of touch or human interaction. Some children live without parents and other adults in the community to care for them. This, too, is the reality of our healthcare world, the place we are in.

Against this backdrop of world reality, we will now, with a quick sweep of a broad brush, characterize the development of ethical theory. In table 1 we identify three periods: traditional, universal, and contingent, built directly from the scholarship of Pellegrino and Gadow. These three periods are characterized in a *linear* way as pre-modern-local, modern-liberal, and post-modern-pluralistic, or, in a *layered* way, as subjective immersion, objective detachment, and intersubjective engagement. One could also see these three periods, in either approach, as unreflective quiescent, active theorizing, and crisis of perspectives. One could think of the questions that might frame the exploration during each of these periods:

- What are you going through?
- What is my duty?
- What virtues do I need?
- What is the goal?
- What is the outcome?
- Who benefits?
  or
- What is fitting?
- What is the right and good thing for me to do?

Or one could think of where attention is directed: to symptomatic description by the person through an interview, to abstract information through observation, or to intersubjective understanding through dialogue. Or, one could see life as

Table 1
Development of Ethical Theory

Ethical Theory	Traditional	Universal	Contingent
Linear	Pre-modern: prior to the 1950s	Modern: from 1950s to 1980-90s	Post-modern: into the 21st century
Layered	Subjective immersion	Objective detachment	Intersubjective engagement
Activity	Unreflective quiescent	Active theorizing	Crisis of perspectives
Focus	Hippocratic Oath	Principles/anti-principles	Relationship
Source	Local	Liberal	Pluralistic
Type of knowledge	Symptomatic	Abstract	Inherent
Approach	Interview	Observation	Dialogue
Questions	What are you going through? What virtues do I need? What is my duty?	What is the goal? What is the outcome? Who benefits?	What is fitting? What is the right and good thing for me to do?
Meaning of life	Life is a mystery.	Life is to be controlled.	Life is to be shared.

a mystery, as something to be controlled, or as something to be shared. Table 1 gives a surface overview of these three periods as if they are distinct. In actual fact, there is considerable overlap.

THE LINEAR VIEW

The linear view of the history of the approaches used in bioethics highlights only areas of development. This depiction is not meant to be a comprehensive historical description, rather it is used as a heuristic device to give a sense as to why we are where we are. *What place are we in?* While Pellegrino uses four periods or eras, we will use three, combining his period of principlism with the period of anti-principlism, as these both fit into what we are calling the universal period. The three linear periods (eras) are the traditional (local) era, the universal (liberal) era, and the contingent (pluralism) era. From the linear perspective, healthcare professionals and philosophers began to study the field of bioethics only in the second period. During the traditional or local era, there was little reflection about matters of ethics.

THE TRADITIONAL (LOCAL) ERA

According to Gadow, the 2,500 years prior to the modern age were a period of "unreflective and uncritical certainty," based on the immersion of the doctor and patient within a family, community, and religious tradition of that time.[31] Doctor and patient both ascribed to the deontological philosophy of the Hippocratic Oath, largely without reflection or analysis. As Pellegrino notes, "Despite the close juxtaposition of medicine and philosophy, the ethic of the Hippocratic corpus never became a subject of formal philosophical scrutiny on its own,"[32] nor was there a treatise on medical ethics produced by philosophers such as Plato, Aristotle, or the Stoics. In fact, according to Pellegrino, the physician-patient relationship was not "systemically justified or derived in any formal way."[33] The certainty of "the good" was understood to come from some outside authority, such as a cultural, professional, or religious belief. Because the community was cohesive in its beliefs and values, there was no need for reflection. When differences in interpretation arose between individuals, the foundational unity that grounded their values prevented differences from becoming divisive.[34] In the early 1900s, both medical and nursing texts emphasized duty, compassion, and the etiquette expected of the "prudent gentleman" and "doctor's handmaiden," the Hippocratic Oath underwent little modification (except to remove traces of pagan origins),[35] and nursing codes of behavior were etiquette-based.[36] Practical wisdom, *phronesis*, guided the physician "to discern the right and good thing to do in the face of a particular moral choice."[37]

The pre-modern period lasted until the middle of the twentieth century, when the Western world experienced a general social upheaval in moral values. With a better-educated public, the spread of participatory democracy (civil rights, patients' rights, and the concept of human rights), feminism, diverse ethnicity, and the rise in science and technology, with its effect to produce good and harm not previously known, there came a heightened distrust of authority and a questioning attitude. The Nazi era, unethical research experiments, and the Trials of War Criminals before the Nuremberg Military Tribunals brought attention to the need for a greater respect of autonomy, policies, and rules about informed consent in clinical practice and in research, and challenges to paternalism that was so much a part of the medical profession.[38] Upheaval in society caused reflection on issues of medical ethics, and lack of certainty in the immediacy of the local tradition-based attitudes of ethics led to an active period of philosophical search for ethical certainty.

THE UNIVERSAL (LIBERAL) ERA

Since the 1950s and 1960s, both philosophers and physicians became committed to finding specific devices that could be used to apply certain moral knowledge to medical practice. This commitment was based on two factors that responded to the turmoil of the age. First, a belief in scientific and philosophical rationality gave physicians and other health-care professionals a strong commitment to, and trust in, expert knowledge, knowledge that gave certainty about how to behave morally. As Pellegrino stated, "Moral philosophy offered a systematic and relatively objective way to approach ethical dilemmas. Its analytic rigor appealed to academic clinicians who were becoming aware of the growing complexity of ethical dilemmas."[39] The desire for certainty in moral knowledge mirrored the expectation for certainty of medical knowledge applied to modern treatment of disease. There was also the increasingly litigious nature of the American public, which enforced a desire for healthcare professionals to know how to behave morally based on philosophically sound and defensible ethical principles.

The second factor that influenced the search for universal certainty in ethics was that philosophers were looking for a place to develop their talents in broader ways. Some philosophers experienced (in twentieth century Anglo-American philosophy) a relatively sterile pursuit in founding all knowledge and practice on the basis of logical principles. Some philosophers realized that this restrictive focus on analytical thought did not provide practical insights for ethics in healthcare. As philosophers were becoming increasingly isolated and removed from practical circumstances, a few seized new developments in applied ethics, specifically medical ethics, as a way to free themselves from the confines of austere philosophical, but less practical, approaches.

These two factors, physicians desiring certainty in moral decision making and philosophers wishing for practical outlets for analytical knowledge, led into a period of active development of philosophical theoretical knowledge in bioethics. According to Gadow, "The modern turn in ethics aims at overcoming the relativity of competing parochial certainties by producing one incontestable system of universal principles."[40] Philosophers brought to bioethics well-established moral traditions, such as deontology, consequentialism, and virtue theory, which had become free of faith commitments. One of the strongest influences in Western bioethics was the "four-principle approach" of Beauchamp and Childress.[41] As Pellegrino noted, "The tetrad of principles had the advantage of being compatible with deontological and consequentialist theories and even with some aspects of virtue theory. It was quickly applied by medical ethicists to resolve ethical dilemmas and was adopted by health professionals."[42]

Numerous challenges to the four-principle approach occurred during these years, such as those raised by Howard

Brody, K. Danner Clouser and Bernard Gert, Tristram Engelhardt, Albert Jonsen, Alasdan MacIntyre, and Edmund
Pellegrino himself.[43] Some thought that principles do not provide adequate directives in actual healthcare situations,[44] lack
sufficient emphasis on care and relationship,[45] ignore the interests of the family,[46] and do not meet some of the needs of
nursing,[47] family medicine,[48] or clinical medicine.[49] The "care"
literature was swelling, and discussion about a justice-care
dichotomy surfaced.[50] Scholars and practitioners questioned
whether an ethics based on the knowledge gained through
science was even possible—a world completely knowable if
just the right tools were used; a world rendered the same for
everyone; a world that was uniform, replicable, and predict-
able. There is an uncomfortable worry that the emphasis on
personal autonomy and self-determination is so necessary precisely because people in social authority (doctors, researchers, et cetera) cannot be trusted.[51] Scholars began to suggest
that other knowledge is needed, based on the assumption that
the world as we live in it (a world that wraps itself around us)
is knowable only to the extent that we share experiences with
each other. As this complex world of contemporary healthcare is experienced, it becomes less certain that rules and principles can provide adequate solutions to ethical dilemmas.[52]

Pellegrino summarizes the challenge to principles as follows: "principles, it is said, are too abstract, too rationalistic,
and too removed from the psychological milieu in which moral
choices are actually made; principles ignore a person's character, life story, cultural background and gender."[53] The concern about principles, indeed the loss of ability to find certainty of knowledge for moral and ethical practice in healthcare, led to a period described as a "crisis" by Pellegrino.
Bauman puts it this way: "moral issues cannot be 'resolved,'
nor the moral life of humanity guaranteed, by the calculating
and legislative efforts of reason. Morality is not safe in the
hands of reason. . . . [Morality needs the] un-founded, non-
rational, un-arguable, no-excuses given and non-calculable
urge to stretch towards the other, to caress, to be for, to live
for, happen what may."[54] A move away from reason and toward each other was heralded by the recognition of the real-

ity of our pluralistic society and the need to find a way to live together by embracing the differences between people.[55]

THE CONTINGENT (PLURALISTIC) ERA

The final period in our discussion of the linear approach to the development of ethical thought began primarily in the 1980s. In the post-modern, pluralistic world, ethical challenges demand not universality, but contingency—a way to connect to the knowledge learned in the tradition-based local and subsequent universal periods. As Pellegrino noted, "What is required is some comprehensive philosophical underpinning for medical ethics that will link the great moral traditions with principles and rules and with the new emphasis on moral psychology. This obviously calls for more than an affable eclecticism."[56] A crisis indicates a need for a turning point or evolution, and it is at this crisis point that we now find ourselves. Pellegrino suggests that one place to turn is to clinical practice—the place where the realities of moral choices are confronted in day-by-day health and medical care. It is to clinical practice, the place of relationship, where we need to focus attention while we continue the dialogue between moral philosophers and healthcare professionals. This time of great turning, precipitated by crisis, is found in many areas of life, not only bioethics, and suggests a need to embrace a dialectic between principles and relationships in our search to nurture moral integrity.[57]

The linear view of the development of bioethics thought and practice is enhanced by a view of these periods as *layered*. Sally Gadow, through an original and unique scholarship, shows how the periods can be seen not only from the view of linear progression but as "elements that coexist in an ethically vital profession."[58] While Gadow uses this approach to build an ethical cornerstone for nursing, her work has the potential to be useful for all health professions.

THE LAYERED VIEW

A linear view seems rather easy to understand—one period of time follows another. With the layered view, Gadow brings history forward in a different and complimentary way—

building on the previous era without losing it in current experience. For example, we need to have subjective, objective, and intersubjective knowledge in current practice. Gadow, building on Hegel's work, develops the layers as necessary results of a dialectical relationship "in which none of the three [layers] can stand alone and only their coexistence constitutes a sound basis for practice."[59] Gadow's original development of the layered dialectic promotes a wonderful way to avoid the dualism of *either/or* and builds ethical scholarship on *both/and.*[60] Through showing the limitations of each layer and responding appropriately, the next layer takes on greater complexity and comprehension. Nothing is lost; everything is attended to, but changed and enhanced in a way that makes for greater usefulness. Gadow shows that the dialectic has a characteristic rhythm of three phases of simplicity, opposition, and reconciliation (thesis-antithesis-synthesis). But, she says, "No phase is exclusively thesis, antithesis, or synthesis. Each phase serves as antithesis of the one before, and each synthesis becomes a new thesis as its own unity is further differentiated."[61] We will now explore the three levels using Gadow's layered approach as another way to see *where we are*: subjective immersion, objective detachment, and intersubjective engagement.

The Level of Subjective Immersion

Gadow describes this early tradition-based era as a less-reflective time in our bioethical history, in which people existed in a cohesive community where uncritical certainty about the good was prevalent. This certainty was found through sources that transcended the individual: religion, family, customs, or the ethos of the profession (particularly medicine). With a cultural, professional, or religious basis for certainty, the healthcare professional and the patient and family intuits the good directly without recourse to reflection.[62] "Immediacy serves to maintain the self—and the group—as a coherent, harmonious whole. Immersion and immediacy, in other words, describe community."[63] Gadow suggests that with the renewed interest in communitarian ethics, there is a move to build ethics on a shared communal interest, which is characteristic of this period. She refers to the communitarian interest to regard individuals as "situated in a natural community such as a family, neighborhood, or nation, a community of origin that anchors personal identity and guarantees moral certainty."[64] Engelhardt's recent text is an ideal example of the communitarian focus of subjective immersion in which moral knowledge is "sustained by a particular moral experience, albeit one of a transcendent God,"[65] based on traditional Christianity of the first millennium. Duty, virtues, and values are governed by the traditional community to which one belongs. When the self and the community are a coherent, harmonious whole, there is no need for personal ethical and moral reflection, as there is no experience of doubt and distress.

Gadow, through dialectic, does not dismiss a tradition-based or communitarian view, but shows its limitations for our current society with its lack of cohesive beliefs, values, and actions. Merely identifying an issue as "ethical" (beginning reflection) undermines immediacy (and its lack of reflectiveness), and results in choice. It is in the notion of choice that the next level is found. If one resists the paternalistic choice of community, religion, or profession, one searches for another form of certainty. Through rational argument of language and reason, one could show why one choice is better than another. Once such questioning and reasoning happens, subjective immediacy is lost and one moves to search for universal knowledge found in objectivity.

The Level of Objective Detachment

Dialectically, the move away from immediacy produces the opposite—rational objectivity—which, as we described above, occurs for numerous reasons. As Gadow noted, at the level of the universal, "rationality counters subjectivity with principles that are categorical and unconditional. Detachment provides the distance needed for objectivity, for viewing from a vantage point outside, instead of inside, the situation."[66] Here, Gadow notes, reason equals universality in the search for "one uncontestable system of universal principles."[67] But, as we have considered above, the search for universal principles has been less successful than originally hoped. Gadow identifies three limitations of the focus on objectivity. First, interpretations of principles can conflict in clinical situations. Second, universalism strips the lived reality of persons and situations and "reduces a professional from an ethical agent to an automaton."[68] Third, ethical universalism is founded on dualism, in which reason is held as the essence of humanness, whereas emotions are seen as unruly, unreliable, and ideally should be ignored. As Gadow notes, "Because universalism values persons as transcendent, it devalues those experiences, already marginalized by dualism, that are not fully controllable, such as illness and suffering. The moral high ground of rationality becomes synonymous with privilege and power instead of the equality it promised."[69] In order to overcome the limitations of the universal level, we need to take a dialectical turn toward a third layer of pluralism and contingency (nondualism), where there is a valuing of persons as irreducibly ambiguous. Here persons are seen as both/and: particular *and* universal, embodied *and* intellectual, emotional *and* rational. The move now is from the detachment of the universal layer to intersubjective engagement.

The Level of Intersubjective Engagement

The turn that is precipitated by crisis (as identified by Pellegrino) is a turn to the uniqueness of persons, each as a *situated self*, a self that encompasses not only rationality but emotion, imagination, memory, language, the body, and cultures. The *situated self* is a relational self, a self that is intersubjective. We are now at the same place where Pellegrino left us in the linear view, a place with a need for "affable eclecticism,"[70] a place where moral choices are confronted in day-to-day health and medical care with real people. Oliver Sacks, a neurologist, says this place is neither subjective nor objective, but is a place where "the physician must proceed by sympathy or empathy, proceeding in company with the patient, *sharing* his experiences and feelings and thoughts, the inner conceptions which shape his behavior. He must feel (or imagine) how his patient is feeling, without ever losing the sense of himself; he must inhabit, simultaneously, two frames of reference, and make it possible for the patient to do likewise."[71] What is so revolutionary about Gadow's dialectical approach to ethical practice for healthcare is her ability to show the three periods not as "successive stages in the profession's advance, but as possibilities coexisting in an ethically vital practice. Dialectic offers a way of envisioning contradictory approaches as intrinsically related. None of the three is fully intelligible without its connection to the others. Each complements the limitations of the other two."[72]

Other scholars have described an ethic that strives to combine these levels (integrating the three periods) that reflects justice and care, with various terms such as nurturance,[73] pedagogical relation,[74] fittingness,[75] moral impulse,[76] quickening,[77] and integrative.[78] In this text, we use the term *relational ethics* to distinguish an approach to ethics that is grounded in practical relations (action-oriented) from approaches that only promote traditional philosophical and bioethical theory (thinking-oriented). We are at a turning point, a crisis, in which we need to return to day-to-day healthcare practice, where one expresses one's commitment to other persons in the ways in which human beings relate to one another.[79]

Lucy van Pelt, from the comic strip "Peanuts," says that she loves humanity but can't stand people. Like Lucy, sometimes it seems easier for us to pay attention to the abstract (humanity) than to enter the complex and often uncomfortable reality of relationships with people day after day (community). The crisis in ethics has turned us toward the need of both objective abstract knowledge (for example, the principle of respect for autonomy) and subjective concrete knowledge (for example, Erika found frozen in the snow). We need both. Consider the following aspects of the current ethical challenge: tensions between the individual and the collective, between autonomy and justice, between participation and omission, between beneficence and equity, and between charity and solidarity. Consider, also, the reality of our world—of poverty, conflict, cultural misunderstandings, healthcare inequities—issues of global injustice. Lastly, consider the world of the wealthy—a world concerned with beginning and end-of-life decision making, issues of resource allocation, and the problems raised by such challenging technologies as cloning and stem cell research—again, issues of social justice.

As we gathered around Erika, we saw the possibility that all levels of knowledge come to the fore. The 911 call by Erika's mother stimulated a number of people whose common goal was to save Erika's life. There was little ethical reflection, as everyone—mother, paramedics, professionals, and technicians—desperately worked toward one goal. Many other resources were also used to work toward this goal. No one acted with doubt or questioning. Saving Erika was the right thing to do. If Erika had been left hovering between life and death, other questions would have been necessary: Is the treatment now contributing to healing or is it preventing a tragic but eventual death? The relational space, the third intersubjective level, is needed for the flow between different types of knowledge (description of symptoms, scientific assessment and treatment, and inherent intersubjective knowledge of human experience). As the world watched in amazement as Erika was brought back to life, we were reminded that all the world's children should be given this same kind of care, through respect for the life of every child, respect for life itself, and provision of enough resources for life to flourish. The relational space would allow asking of the difficult questions about how children need safe, supervised places and adequate clothing, even as they sleep. Perhaps the relational space can provide a "container" for interactions between people and ideas, between theory and practice. Such a container could also provide space for reflection and integration.[80]

BUILDING A RELATIONAL ETHIC

Gadow uses the image of a coral reef—new generations built on the residue of the old—to illustrate how different forms of knowledge can live together so that ethical knowledge can continue to develop. None of the knowledge developed during the various periods of history of Western bioethics can be dismissed. Rather, there is a need for knowledge to be integrated, so that more complex and more comprehensive knowledge can be created. Western bioethics also needs to consider, discuss, and value bioethics approaches learned from other cultures.[81] Like a coral reef, all previous forms of knowledge remain as supporting structure for new life and growth. Gadow says, "at the level of immediacy, we are immersed in ethical currents that carry us safely through situations where reflection would be impossible. When crosscurrents require us to reflect and to hold a position, an edifice of ethical principles offers a structure for steadying ourselves. Finally, there are situations where no edifice can alleviate our vulnerability, and in those cases we can only turn to each other and together compose a fragile new form of the good."[82]

Another image, a bountiful tree with roots and branches, gives a sense of the importance and usefulness of a relational ethic. The trunk of the tree holds the space that integrates branches and roots. The trunk of a tree is not a space *between* the branches and roots but is *integral* to both, as neither branches nor roots can live without the other. The trunk is the relational space that supports the flow between branches and roots. Like the other polarities of our current life (subjective and objective, experience and science, self and other) there is a need to attend to the reality of the space, the tree trunk, to support the flow between these oppositions. It is in practical life, like the living tree, where oppositions cease. Often, in life, the tree trunk is not considered (other than its height), as one naturally goes to the fruit and the leaves, or to the gnarled roots (visible and deeper) that anchor the tree. Yet, in life, the trunk is the vital nurturing power. If one is situated in one or the other, branches or roots, life is not lived to its fullest. If one identifies only with the branches (objectivity), one loses the nourishment of the roots (subjectivity). If one lives only through the branches (the rational mind), one misses the wisdom of the roots (the lived body), and wholeness is lost. In the same way, if one is caught only in matter (body, the earth, the valley) one loses the clarity and perspective of the spirit (thinking mind, the sky, the top of the mountain). If one is caught in either pole, unnatural death occurs. If one lives in wholeness (branches, trunk, and roots) death will still come, but it has the potential to come with more grace and acceptance. The dynamic trunk (relationship) is essential for an ethical life to flourish.

Pellegrino and Gadow have shown us where we are, and we now begin to describe this place more fully. Our task in this text is to reveal a relational space (the trunk of the tree) that is integrative and living. In each of the subsequent chapters, we focus on an identified theme for a relational ethic to flourish: mutual respect, engaged interaction, embodiment, and interdependent environment where freedom and choice are found. We know from experience that relational ethics (using all levels and approaches to ethical knowledge) is practiced and present in our healthcare world, yet there is need to give it particular attention and language. Such a language would express complex views of harmony, community, and sustainability that are more comprehensive and productive than our current focus.[83]

As you read the following chapters, you will notice within each theme consistent threads that run through the text: what it means to be a person, the importance and commitment to community, and the ongoing need to "live in the questions." These threads provide the structure for this action-oriented dynamic relational ethic to flourish as a living entity. When Raymond Duff says, "the secret of caring for the patient is caring for the patient,"[84] he is giving voice to that relational place, the ethical moment where people connect with each other. This moment of practice can be full of activity, or it can be full of stillness. Not a stillness that leaves patients and families bereft, but a stillness that means *being with* each other. Practice, as action, means more than just doing something, such as an active intervention (or treatment to effect a cure). Sometimes action means *just* being there: "Don't just do something, stand there!" Be there. Be with the other.

A recent nonfiction Dutch film, *Death on Request*, brings the ethics of practice clearly to light.[85] In the film, Kees van Wendel de Joode, who has progressive amyotrophic lateral sclerosis (ALS—Lou Gehrig's disease) requests that the family doctor, Van Oijen, assist him to die when he decides that life is no longer bearable. The film shows the process of decision making by Kees, Antoinette (his wife), and the doctor, to the point of Kees's death. The dialogue about euthanasia is raised throughout this real-life drama between Kees and Antoinette, Kees and the doctors, Antoinette and Van Oijen, and with other professionals. The question of euthanasia is acted out in all the activities leading to the death; a death described as right, peaceful, and beautiful by Kees's wife. The tragedy of the experience is present throughout. Logical thinking, touch, emotion, and pain are all there. This film does not lead us through a theoretical discussion of euthanasia; rather, it shows the ongoing struggle to meet the needs of another human being faced with a tragic life experience. It shows that ethics is a constant questioning, with ongoing dialogue for Kees, for Antoinette, and for Dr. Oijen. It shows the need for all forms of knowledge—the experiences of all the people involved, the clinical knowledge of the deteriorating health of Kees, and the ongoing discussion these people had together. At the end of the film the question of euthanasia remains—as it should. Ethics of practice leads to the ongoing ethical dialogue of how to be more human.[86] The place we are in is one of relation to both self and other that gives place to being a person, fostering community, and living the questions.

BEING A PERSON: AUTONOMY IN RELATION

In the world of practice—as well as in the world of theory—autonomy and self-determination are vitally important. In practice, we see how autonomy is lived in relation to others. Autonomy, as lived, is a relational experience that involves both independence from others and dependence on others. As a *lived concept*, autonomy is understood as an interdependent notion. While the principle of respect for autonomy has been important in the development of human rights as self-determination and personal freedom, the concept of lived autonomy is found in personal connection to others and responsibility. Autonomy is developed over a lifetime and is not a goal that is reached once and for all time. An overemphasis on autonomy as a right (individual, racial, or religious) can lead to intolerance, and, perhaps more significantly, to a lack of responsibility for and connection to others. An overemphasis on autonomy leads to a life in which everyone fends for the self. *Self-in-relation* is a notion that considers the complexity of who we are as persons: with depth, both independent and dependent; with both individual rights and interdependent responsibilities; and with both intellectual abilities and emotional ties.

Human beings are interdependent whole persons, social beings by design, not choice. As Raymond Duff noted, "We constantly take others into ourselves and give to others in return [and must understand ourselves in the social context of] how we live together."[87] Instead of "I think, therefore I am," a relational approach may hold the premise, "I am, because of you," or "I am because we are."[88] Many scholars (particularly environmentalists) extend the notion of interdependency to include all life, not just human social relations. The work of *deep bioethics* highlights the need for broad ecological considerations for health ethics.[89] Another example of interdependedness research in genetics reminds us of our bodily connection to others in families and relationships. Genetic information is different from other personal information, as it tells, not just a personal story, but a story that includes everyone else to whom one is related. As both personal and familial, genetic information places the notion of privacy and relationality in the foreground. It raises questions of our moral commitment to both self and others at the same time.[90] While genetic information is just one kind of information, it does show the reality of our connection to others. Interdependency is our human reality.

Within an interdependent world reality, being a person is not limited to the disembodied, rational, autonomous, separate, isolated, and abstract articulation of personhood, as it is sometimes often conceived. Rather, personhood is built on the premise that, as John Macmurray stated, "human experience is, in principle, shared experience," which leads us to understand ourselves, as persons, not as an "I" but as a "You and I."[91] Often in healthcare, autonomy is thought to equal personal choice and independence. But that notion of autonomy is an oversimplification of the moral ideal of self-governance, says Susan Sherwin.[92] Autonomy is not a static state achieved by virtue of achieving adulthood, but is a dynamic process of self-discovery through interaction with others. This conception of person allows maturity to include dependence as well as independence, where both dependence and independence exist equally well in an interdependent reality. The notion of person as relational speaks to Bauman's notion of "the moral party of two,"[93] the connections that bind us together as humans. We are not alone and can never be alone. We experience loneliness precisely because we are interdependent.

Within this reality of interdependence, we need to reconsider the expectation that maturity equals independence alone. We have come to believe that, developmentally, we move from dependence as a child to independence as an adult. However, within an interdependent notion, the child moves from interdependence as a child to interdependence as an adult. "Person as relation" challenges the principle of autonomy, the idea that a person can stand completely alone. Rather, recognition and acceptance of interrelationships between persons as the ground of morality makes possible the freedom of all.[94] Thus, freedom for all members of a society depends upon the notion of the shared interdependency of each with the other, where relationality and individuality are essential dimensions or "poles" of personhood. Neither individuality or relationality, of themselves, constitute a person's total reality, as a person does not stand completely alone, nor is a person reduced to a web of relations. Each person has personal identity and individuality, yet, as Walter Jeffko reminds us, "relationality is primary and individuality is secondary, in the sense that persons are constituted as individual persons within the inclusive field of persons-in-relation."[95]

When one is involved in the daily action of caring for another (as nurse-patient, doctor-patient, midwife-woman, or care attendant-chronically ill person), one travels with the other as if on a journey. Sharing experiences, feelings, and thoughts and using imagination to understand another's pain contributes to a relation that blurs the sharp distinction between professionals and patients that is so important to the current ethical framework. Yet a relational perspective does not mean that one loses the sense of self nor the opportunity for self-determination. Rather, in spite of the confusion and the shifting of boundaries, each person may come to experience the self and the other more clearly through the honest effort to keep conversation open.

FOSTERING COMMUNITY:
SITUATING OURSELVES IN DIALOGUE

To move past the dichotomy of micro issues versus macro issues, it is helpful to reconstruct another view of community. In a society that has become increasingly fragmented, where we have diversity without unity and the assertion of individual rights without a vision of responsibility for the larger community, we need to consider a new way of thinking about community. Jeffko, following John Macmurray, suggests a principle or standard called *community* that could be the paramount ethical principle.[96] "Since the field of morality is the field of interpersonal action and relations, the principle of community considers the good or well-being—what Macmurray calls the 'harmony'—of each and every person, in both their relational and their individual aspects."[97] How a person is treated and treats oneself has moral significance. Jeffko's principle of community describes "an action as morally right if it promotes a personal relation of persons, either interpersonal or intrapersonal, and it is morally wrong if it directly intends an absolute impersonal relation of persons."[98] Impersonal relations between persons occur when people are treated in an instrumental way (for example, as an object, a disease, a role, or a means to an end). Personal relations are those in which people are treated and valued as whole persons. A community standard or principle holds that the good (flourishing) of both self and other as primary, so that all people are valued for themselves.

The emerging pluralism, with its embrace of difference, is proving unsettling and unnerving, as we no longer are absolutely sure who is at the center and who is at the margins, who is a neighbor and who is the stranger, who are "we" and who are "they."[99] Our landscape is changing so much that there is no immunity from exclusion. Such a pluralistic reality calls us to embrace difference—difference between ourselves and others and the difference that we find within ourselves. It means coming face-to-face with people who are different, but without self-effacement on our part or debasement on the part of the other. Community is achieved and maintained through ethical action of deep and full respect for ourselves and our neighbors, friends, and enemies, as persons. This notion of community is very different from a communitarian view, where we all think alike. Here we value community through respecting, indeed embracing, difference, and, in doing so, strive to dissolve the we/they duality by holding the space/

relationship between. Communitarian views build on agreement of similar values and work from that consensus of sameness. Communitarian views always encounter we/they. Community asks us to talk together—mutually—in spite of our differences.

"Morality is rooted in collective life," says Daniel Chambliss; "ethical problems in healthcare are inseparable from the organizational and social setting in which they arise."[100] But human society, as a unity of persons, is not merely a matter of fact, but a matter of intention. "We have the capacity to imagine a better future," said George Erasmus, "and we have the tools at hand."[101] We just need to act. The crisis in ethics invites a turning of attention to the broader issues of our collective life and to recognize the links between ecological ethics and medical ethics, between the rights for individual autonomy and the needs and survival of community, and between the need for science to focus on molecular genetics and the need for focus on ecological sciences.[102] To be ethical in practice we need to pay attention to developing a common intention. If that intention is to promote the deep and complex relations of persons in healthcare situations, the impact is enormous.

LIVING THE QUESTIONS: LETTING GO OF SURENESS

If the moral rightness of action has its ground in the relations of persons, as Macmurray asserts, then "the moral problematic of all action—the possibility that any action may be morally right or wrong—arises from the conflict of wills, and morality, in any mode, is the effort to resolve this conflict."[103] Resolving conflicts or considering ethical dilemmas has most often been addressed by a problem-solving approach, which is characteristic of the modernist desire for certainty. Often ethical dilemmas are attempted to be solved by a problem-solving approach with the following steps:
1. Describe the problem,
2. Gather the facts,
3. Clarify values,
4. Note reactions,
5. Identify ethical principles,

6. Clarify legal rules,
7. Explore options and alternatives,
8. Decide a course of action,
9. Develop an action plan,
10. Act on the plan, and
11. Re-evaluate the whole process.[104]

Another approach to resolving, or perhaps "dis-solving," ethical conflicts might be to ask questions that relate to the experience of people involved in the confusion or dilemma, such as: *What are you going through? How can I understand your experience?* or *What is the best thing (the most fitting) to do, in this situation?*

Robert Burch states that there are four differences when one focuses attention on *questions* instead of *problems*.[105] First, when the focus is on problems, the concern is on "objects" that can be dealt with using implements, concepts, or cognition, whereas, when the focus is on questions, we are concerned with the ways in which we are in the situation, and we do not have the certainty that problem-solving suggests. "We do not so much posit a question, as we are encompassed by it, we do not so much *have* a question, as we *are* in it," says Burch.[106] Second, when we focus on problems, we attack these problems by methods that conquer and provide closure, using abstraction, calculation, and exactness, whereas the use of questions can be revealing, disclosive, integrative, evocative, and open-ended in nature, and can lead to self-appropriation and self-understanding. Third, solving problems is a matter of cognition and control (and mistakes are the opposite of correctness), whereas the use of questions concerns the elucidation of meaning, which encompasses a global set of interpretive horizons. Lastly, answering problems concerns what we do (deploying the objective realm of theoretical, scientific, and practical activities), whereas responding to questions concerns who we are as human beings. Burch says, "it is we ourselves, our having and doing, thinking and being together, that is the principal matter at issue."[107]

Relational ethics does not discard the problem-solving approach to ethical dilemmas, but encourages the reflective approach of asking questions of the human meanings that are encompassed in real life problems. It is in this mode of questioning—of asking who we are—that the theme of relationships is grounded. The heart of relational ethics is ongoing questioning: *What should we do, now?* or *Are we sure?* If ethics is a matter of nurturing questions[108] instead of depending on normative definitions or conclusive answers, then it requires deliberation, self-questioning, uncertainty, and contemplation: *Did I think of everything? Did I do the right thing there? What were the steps taken to make that decision? What was my logic?* We may wonder: *Is this the way I want to live my life? Is this the kind of life I want for my children? Is this the kind of life I want for others? Are you sure? Am I sure?* In most healthcare professions, ethical questioning is a daily activity. As was noted during an IRG session,

> *Perhaps it could be called a "street talk" ethic. I can imagine that in the coffee room someone would say, "What are we doing? It's crazy. Can't we ever give up? I wish someone would really go in and talk to him. But he is a really difficult patient to look after." So that's street talk. For the most part, the problem gets solved there—at that level of day-to-day interaction, and not with everyone sitting down and getting a clipboard and going through the principles— maleficience, beneficence. . . .*[109]

Sometimes it is important to make compare little "e" ethics (everyday practice, how we show respect, the consent process, et cetera) with big "E" ethics (euthanasia, reproductive technologies, the genome project, et cetera). But at the level of practice, the distinction loses its meaning for the root of the question is the same: *How should you and I be treated?*

CONCLUSION

In this chapter, we have developed the place of relational ethics within the context of the development of knowledge about bioethics. Of course, as a cursory history, it is only valuable as a heuristic device to situate us in the development of the field of health ethics. It shows how an ethical focus on relationship is timely and necessary for health ethics to flourish in our pluralistic world. In such a world, we need to come to a better understanding of how to live well, together, in everyday ways. It is not surprising that the story of a baby, a baby like Erika Nordby, captures our attention. Not only are we amazed that she was brought back to life, but we are amazed that many children around the world die in equally dramatic circumstances, that and very few of us notice. The old methods of ethical thinking are not working for the good of all.

The old methods of competition, individual rights, and dominance of the rich are not working. We need a new ethic. Where can we learn this new ethic? Perhaps we need to reflect on early historical stories (myths, legends, stories from various religions, and so on). The biblical story of Adam, Eve, and the snake in the Garden of Eden is one such story. It is an instructive story of autonomy and relationship. It is a story of freedom. Eve and Adam, in eating the fruit, chose knowledge and freedom to make their own decisions (autonomy) about how to live. They chose to be with each other, to know each other, to desire each other, and to have children (relationships). The story of freedom, is a story of autonomy and relationship. It is a life that fosters autonomy through relationships with one another. It is a life that supports freedom and reminds us of the choices we make in living with each other.

We will now move into exploring themes of a relational approach to ethics. In chapter three, we begin exploring the core and fundamental element of mutual respect that includes respect for self as well as for others.

NOTES

1. Edmund Pellegrino, "The Metamorphosis of Medical Ethics: A 30-Year Retrospective," *Journal of the American Medical Association* 269, no. 9 (1993): 1158-62.

2. Charles Taylor, *Philosophy and the Human Sciences*, vol. 2 of *Philosophical Papers* (New York: Cambridge University Press, 1985).

3. A.C. McIntyre, *After Virtue: A Study in Moral Theory*, 2nd ed. (Notre Dame, Ind.: University of Notre Dame Press, 1984).

4. Susan Sherwin, *No Longer Patient: Feminist Ethics and Health Care* (Philadelphia: Temple University Press, 1992); Claudia Card, ed., *Feminist Ethics* (Lawrence, Kans.: University

Press of Kansas, 1991); Rosemarie Tong, "The Ethics of Care: A Feminist Virtue Ethics of Care for Healthcare Practitioners," *Journal of Medicine and Philosophy* 23, no. 2 (1998): 131-52.

5. Annette Baier, "What Do Women Want in a Moral Theory?" *Nous* 19 (1985): 53-63; Alisa Carse, "The 'Voice of Care': Implications for Bioethics Education," *Journal of Medicine and Philosophy* 16, no. 1 (1991): 5-28; Carol Gilligan, *In a Different Voice: Psychological Theory and Women's Development* (Cambridge, Mass.: Harvard University Press, 1982); Nel Noddings, *Caring: A Feminine Approach to Ethics and Moral Education* (Berkeley, Calif.: University of California Press, 1984).

6. Albert R. Jonsen and Stephen Toulmin, *The Abuse of Casuistry: A History of Moral Reasoning* (Berkeley, Calif.: University of California Press, 1988).

7. Ruth Groenhout, "The Virtue of Care: Aristotelian Ethics and Contemporary Ethics of Care," in *Feminist Interpretations of Aristotle*, ed. Cynthia A. Freeland (University Park, Pa.: Pennsylvania State University Press, 1998).

8. Raanon Gillon, ed., *Principles of Health Care Ethics* (New York: John Wiley & Sons, 1994), 691.

9. Ruth Macklin, "Ethical Relativism in a Multicultural Society," *Kennedy Institute of Ethics Journal* 8, no. 1 (1998): 1-22.

10. See note 1 above.

11. Tom L. Beauchamp and James F. Childress, *Principles of Biomedical Ethics*, 4th ed. (New York: Oxford University Press, 1994).

12. Baruch A. Brody, "Quality of Scholarship in Bioethics," *Journal of Medicine and Philosophy* 15, no. 2 (1990): 161-78.

13. For example, see Annette Baier, "The Need for More than Justice," *Canadian Journal of Philosophy* 13 (1987): 41-55; Walter G. Jeffko, *Contemporary Ethical Issues: A Personalistic Perspective* (Amherst, N.Y.: Humanity Books, 1999); Adriaan Theodoor Peperzak, *Before Ethics* (Amherst, N.Y.: Humanity Books, 1998); J. Nedelsky, ed., *Feminist Theory* (Toronto, Ont.: Faculty of Law, University of Toronto, 1990).

14. Gilligan, see note 5 above.

15. For example: Noddings, see note 5 above; and Baier, see note 13 above.

16. Carol Gilligan, "Remapping the Moral Domain: New Images of Self in Relationship," in *Mapping the Moral Domain: A Contribution of Women's Thinking to Psychological Theory and Education*, ed. C. Gilligan et al. (Cambridge, Mass.: Harvard Uni-

versity Press, 1988), 35, 47.

17. Robin S. Dillon, "Respect and Care: Toward Moral Integration," *Canadian Journal of Philosophy* 22, no. 1 (1992): 105-32; Virginia Held, "The Meshing of Care and Justice," *Hypatia* 10, no. 2 (1995): 128-32.

18. Baier, see note 13 above, p. 44.

19. Wilf Backhaus, "Shaking the Pillars: Quality and Unspoken Bioethical Values in a Pluralistic Society," in *Quality Culture: Quality in Turbulent Times*, ed. J. Ross et al. (Camrose, Alb.: J. Ross Enterprises, 1994).

20. Robert A. Burt, *Taking Care of Strangers: The Rule of Law in Doctor-Patient Relations* (New York: Free Press, 1979), 101.

21. Richard Gelwick, "The Patient Self-Determination Act and 'Dax's Case'," *Journal of Medical Humanities* 13, no. 3 (1992): 177-87; Gilbert Meilaender, "Reconciling Rights and Responsibilities: Our Vocabularies, Our Selves," *Hastings Center Report* 24, no. 3 (1994), 13-4.

22. Meilaender, see note 21 above, p. 14.

23. Zygmunt Bauman, *Postmodern Ethics* (Oxford, U.K.: Blackwell, 1993).

24. Mary Ann Glendon, *Rights Talk: The Impoverishment of Political Discourse* (New York: Free Press, 1991).

25. Sally Gadow, "Relational Narratives: The Postmodern Turn in Nursing Ethics," *Scholarly Inquiry for Nursing Practice: An International Journal* 13, no. 1 (1999): 57-70.

26. Robert Helmich Henson, "Analysis of the Concept of Mutuality," *Image: Journal of Nursing Scholarship* 29, no. 1 (1997): 77-81.

27. Held, see note 17 above, p. 132.

28. See note 1 above.

29. See note 25 above.

30. Chris Purdy, "Saving a Frozen Girl," *Edmonton Journal*, 25 February 2001, A1; Chris Purdy, "A Baby Named 'Miracle'," *Edmonton Journal*, 26 February 2001, A1; Chris Purdy, "Erika's Mom Blames Herself for Mishap," *Edmonton Journal*, 28 February 2001, A1, A10.

31. See note 25 above, p. 59.

32. See note 1 above, p. 1159.

33. Ibid.

34. See note 25 above.

35. See note 1 above. See chapter seven for further discussion of professional codes.

36. American Nurses Association, "A Suggested Code: A Code of Ethics Presented for the Consideration of the American Nurses' Association," *American Journal of Nursing* 26 (1926): 599-601; American Nurses Association, "A Tentative Code: For the Nursing Profession," *American Journal of Nursing* 40 (1940): 977-80; M. Cianci, "The Code of Ethics and the Role of Nurses: An Historical Perspective," *Nursing Connections* 5, no. 1 (1992): 37-42; L. Freitas, "Historical Roots and Future Perspectives Related to Nursing Ethics," *Journal of Professional Nursing* 6, no. 4 (1990): 197-205.

37. See note 1 above, p. 1159.

38. Robert A. Burt, "The Suppressed Legacy of Nuremberg," *Hastings Center Report* 26, no. 5, (1996): 30-3.

39. See note 37 above.

40. See note 25 above, p. 61.

41. Tom L. Beauchamp and James F. Childress, *Principles of Biomedical Ethics*, 1st ed. (New York: Oxford University Press, 1979).

42. See note 1 above, p. 1160.

43. Challenges to principlism have been put forth by: Brody, see note 12 above; K. Danner Clouser and Bernard Gert, "A Critique of Principlism," *Journal of Medicine and Philosophy* 15, no. 2 (1990): 219-36; H. Tristram Englehardt, *The Foundations of Bioethics* (New York: Oxford University Press, 1986); H. Tristram Englehardt and Michael A. Rie, "Morality for the Medical-Industrial Complex: A Code of Ethics for the Mass Marketing of Health Care," *New England Journal of Medicine* 319, no. 16 (1988): 1086-9; Jonsen and Toulmin, see note 6 above; Alasdair MacIntyre, "A Crisis in Moral Philosophy: Why Is the Search for Foundations so Frustrating?" in *Knowing and Valuing: The Search for Common Roots*, ed. H. Tristram Englehardt and Daniel Callahan (Hastings-on-Hudson, N.Y.: Hastings Center, 1980), 18-33; Pellegrino, see note 1 above.

44. Terrence Ackerman, "Medical Ethics and the Two Dogmas of Liberalism," *Theoretical Medicine* 5, no. 1 (1984): 69-81; Clouser and Gert, "A Critique of Principlism," see note 43 above; Robert L. Holmes, "The Limited Relevance of Analytical Ethics to the Problems of Bioethics," *Journal of Medicine and Philosophy* 15, no. 2 (1990): 143-59; Stephen Toulmin, "The Tyranny of Principles," *Hastings Center Report* 11, no. 6 (1981): 31-9.

45. Gilligan, see note 5 above; see note 16 above.

46. John Hardwig, "What about the Family?" *Hastings Cen-*

64 *Relational Ethics*

ter Report 20, no. 2 (1990), 5-10.

47. M.C. Cooper, "Reconceptualizing Nursing Ethics . . . Including Commentary by M.J. Watson," *Scholarly Inquiry for Nursing Practice* 4, no. 3 (1990): 209-21; Sara Fry, "The Role of Caring in a Theory of Nursing Ethics," *Hypatia* 4, no. 2 (1989): 88-103.

48. Ronald J. Christie and C. Barry Hoffmaster, *Ethical Issues in Family Medicine* (New York: Oxford University Press, 1986).

49. Richard M. Zaner, *Ethics and the Clinical Encounter* (Englewood Cliffs, N.J.: Prentice Hall, 1988).

50. Cooper, see note 47 above; Fry, "The Role of Caring," see note 47 above; Sally Gadow, "Response to 'Personal Knowing: Evolving Research and Practice'," *Scholarly Inquiry for Nursing Practice* 4, no. 2 (1990): 167-70.

51. See note 38 above.

52. Cooper, see note 47 above.

53. See note 1 above, p. 1161.

54. See note 23 above, p. 247.

55. James H. Olthuis, ed., *Towards an Ethic of Community: Negotiations of Difference in a Pluralist Society* (Waterloo, Ont.: Wilfrid Laurier University Press, 2000).

56. See note 1 above, p. 1161.

57. Joanna Macy and Molly Young Brown, *Coming Back to Life* (Gabriola Island, B.C.: New Society Publishers, 1998).

58. See note 25 above, p. 57.

59. Ibid., 58.

60. Dialectic is accomplished when an ideational entity is transformed into its opposite, and is preserved and fulfilled by it, the combination of the two revealing a higher form of truth. Gadow has developed the dialectic in a number of papers worthy of investigation. These include: Sally Gadow, "Existential Ecology: The Human/Natural World," *Social Science and Medicine* 35, no. 4 (1992): 597-602; and Sally Gadow, "The Dialectic of Clinical Judgment," in *Clinical Judgment: A Critical Appraisal*, ed. H.Tristram Englehardt, Stuart F. Spicker, and Bernard Towers (Dordrecht, the Netherlands: D. Reidel, 1979), 248-53.

61. See note 25 above, p. 59.

62. See note 25 above.

63. Ibid., 60.

64. Ibid., 59. In this quotation, Gadow is paraphrasing the ideas of McIntyre, see note 3 above.

65. H.Tristram Englehardt, *The Foundations of Christian Bioethics* (Lisse, the Netherlands: Swets & Zeitlinger, 2000), xviii.

66. See note 25 above, p. 61.

67. Ibid., 61.
68. Ibid., 62.
69. Ibid.
70. See note 1 above, p. 1161.
71. Oliver Sacks, *Awakenings* (New York: Harper Perennial, 1973 and 1990), 226.
72. See note 25 above, p. 66.
73. Sandra McKinnon, "Nurturance: An Exploration of the Concept" (unpublished paper, University of Alberta, Edmonton, Alb., 1993).
74. Max van Manen, "Vitality of the Pedagogical Relation," in *Reflections on Pedagogy and Method*, vol. 2 (Utrecht, the Netherlands: Proceedings of the University of Utrecht International Pedagogy Conference, 1992), 173-92.
75. R. Melvin Keiser, *Roots of Relational Ethics: Responsibility in Origin and Maturity in H. Richard Niebuhr* (Atlanta, Ga.: Scholars Press, 1996).
76. See note 23 above.
77. Vangie Bergum, *A Child on Her Mind: The Experience of Becoming a Mother* (Westport, Conn.: Bergin & Garvey, 1997).
78. Robert Lyman Potter, "On Our Way to Integrated Bioethics: Clinical/Organizational/Communal," *The Journal of Clinical Ethics* 10, no. 3 (1999): 171-7.
79. Myra Levine, "Nursing Ethics and the Ethical Nurse," *American Journal of Nursing* 7 (1977): 845-9.
80. The notion of *container* was brought to the author's attention by Kris Lund, a doctoral student in theology at the University of Alberta in August 2001.
81. Godfrey B. Tangwa, "The Traditional African Perception of a Person," *Hastings Center Report* 30, no. 5 (2000): 39-43.
82. See note 25 above, p. 66.
83. Peter Whitehouse, "Bioethics, Biology, the Biosphere: The Ecomedical Disconnection Syndrome," *Hastings Center Report* 29, no. 1 (1999): 41-4.
84. Raymond Duff, " 'Close-up' versus 'Distant' Ethics: Deciding the Care of Infants with Poor Prognosis," *Seminars in Perinatology* 11, no. 3 (1987): 244-53, 245.
85. Maarten Nederhorst, *Death on Request*, VHS (Amsterdam: the Netherlands: First Run/Icarus Films/Fanlight Productions, 1994). This example was used in a previous publication by Vangie Bergum. See Vangie Bergum, "Ethics as Question," in *Extending the Boundaries of Care: Medical Ethics & Caring Practices*, ed. Tamara Kohn and Rosemary McKechnic (Oxford, U.K.: Berg Pub-

lishers, 1999).

86. Jean Grondin, *Sources of Hermeneutics* (Albany, N.Y.: State University of New York Press, 1995).

87. See note 84 above, p. 244.

88. Kris Lund, conversation with authors, August 2001; Gillon, see note 8 above.

89. See note 83 above.

90. Lori d'Agincourt-Canning, "Genetic Testing for Hereditary Cancer: Support for a Relational View of Autonomy," (paper presented at the annual meeting of the Canadian Bioethics Society, Edmonton, Alb., October 1999).

91. John Macmurray, *Persons in Relation*, vol. 2 of *The Form of the Personal* (London, U.K.: Faber & Faber, 1961), 61.

92. Susan Sherwin, ed., *The Politics of Women's Health: Exploring Agency and Autonomy* (Philadelphia: Temple University Press, 1998).

93. See note 23 above.

94. See note 91 above.

95. Jeffko, see note 13 above, p. 4.

96. Ibid.

97. Ibid., 21.

98. Ibid., 22.

99. James Olthuis, *Knowing Other-wise: Philosophy at the Threshold of Spirituality* (New York: Fordham University Press, 1997); see note 55 above.

100. Daniel F. Chambliss, *Beyond Caring: Hospital, Nurses, and the Social Organization of Ethics* (Chicago: University of Chicago Press, 1996), 185, 182.

101. George Erasmus, "Why Can't We Talk?" (Toronto) *Globe and Mail*, 9 March 2002, F6-7.

102. See note 78 above; Van Rensselaer Potter, "Aldo Leopold's Land Ethic Revisited: Two Kinds of Bioethics," *Perspectives in Biology and Medicine* 30, no. 2 (1987): 157-69; see note 81 above.

103. See note 91 above, p. 116.

104. Margaret Keatings and O'Neil B. Smith, *Ethical and Legal Issues in Canadian Nursing* (Toronto: W.B. Saunders, 1995), 105-6.

105. Robert Burch, "Confronting Technophobia: A Topology," *Phenomenology + Pedagogy* 4, no. 2 (1986): 3-21.

106. Ibid., 6-7.

107. Ibid., 7.

108. Bergum, see note 85 above.

109. Interdisciplinary Research Group #4.

3

Mutual Respect

INTRODUCTION

In this chapter, and throughout this book, we describe how important philosophical and practical knowledge of healthcare ethics is focussed on the *relationship* itself. The nature of healthcare ethics, from the perspective of the relationships that occur in practice, yields possibilities for right action to be discovered and grasped through conversation, reflection, and commitment. When we focus on relationships, with a goal of human flourishing, ethical questions such as *How should I act?* turn attention not only to *what* we do, but also to *who* we are. Who we are has to do with respect, respect for self and respect for others.

In *The Ethical Demand*, Knud Løgstrup says that it is our attitudes toward one another that help to shape each other's world: "We can make it large or small, bright or drab, rich or dull, threatening or secure. We help shape his world not by theories and views but by our attitude towards him."[1] It became clear early in our research experience, in using a method based on collaborative dialogue between healthcare practitioners and scholars from different disciplines, that *respect for one another* is an essential aspect of a relational ethic. Different disciplines, different genders, different access to power, and different knowledge(s) are present in all healthcare relations and are embodied on any interdisciplinary team, including patients. These differences need to be acknowledged and valued. Recognition of the uniqueness of varied skills and roles (medical, nursing, patient, and legal), varied orientations (theological, psychological, anthropological, and philosophical), and diverse backgrounds (culture, gender, race, and ability) attune us to the need to attend to the differences between people and the necessity of acknowledging and appreciating difference. But respect for difference (for example, power, knowledge, beliefs and values, experience, attitude) does not come easily. Perhaps the most difficult concept for healthcare professionals is that, in *mutual* respect, the professional's self is as important, yet not more important, as those who are cared for.

How does one perceive respect? How does power (in terms of expertise or academic qualifications) or the attributes of individual powerful persons (seasoned scholars versus students, men versus women, doctors versus nurses, healthcare workers versus patients) limit and control the kind of issues that are discussed and the observations that are made? How do patients and families perceive respectfulness? Can we treat everyone equally and still treat everyone uniquely? Respect cannot be ordered by saying "You must be respectful of others." How, then, can mutual respect be understood?

The word *respect* has a number of definitions. One can show respect (consideration), give respect (honor, esteem), be respectful (deference), have self-respect (a felt self-worthiness), provide respectful acknowledgment (regard, love), give respectful distance (allow personal space and privacy), or stand in silent respect (honoring the dead). Within these and other myriad ways of thinking about respect, the sense of *worth* or *worthiness* seems to be at the heart and core of contemporary notions of respect, including self-respect.[2] *Mutual* respect includes both being respectful to self and being respectful of others, and, as such, includes respect *from* others (for example, the midwife respects the birthing woman, and the woman respects the midwife). The word *mutual* directs attention to the interactive and reciprocal nature of respect. It seems easy to speak of respect, "I respect your wish for . . . " yet harder to practice the attitude of "I respect you," especially if I think what you do is inappropriate. Sometimes we hear, or might even say, "Any self-respecting person [mother, father, son, or daughter] would never . . . ," or "I respect this person but . . . " which seems like using the idea of *respect* in an attitude of power or using the word *respect* in a disrespectful way.

In this chapter, we will explore mutual respect by using the story of K'aila[3] as an example and by placing his story within a world where connections to one another are given attention. In such an interdependent world, every person is understood to be a part of the whole, and every person affects and is affected by every other person. We will develop the notion of *personhood* as a concept that is experienced through relationships with others. With mutual respect, we make the distinction between fostering autonomy, as a living, active notion, and respect for autonomy, as a theoretical, abstract construct. The Indo-European root of the word respect, *spek,* means "to regard or to look again," while the Latin *spex* refers to "he who sees."[4] These roots point to the attention that is needed to respect—attention to look again and to actually *see* the other. But it is not just the other who needs attention. In mutual respect, one needs to attend to the self as well. As more than one person is involved in mutual respect, there is an implied symmetry in relationship in terms of acknowledgment, valuing, and the worthiness of each other. One wonders if mutual respect can occur in a situation in which one does not like the other person. Can one empathize and still be appalled? This chapter will close by discussing the potential of mutual respect to address issues of power and how mutual respect can put power in its proper place.

AUTONOMY IN RELATIONSHIP

Mutual respect occurs in an atmosphere of interdependence, where I acknowledge that what I do affects you, and what you do affects me.[5] Interdependence incorporates the view that "*my* freedom depends on how *you* behave."[6] We will use the story of K'aila to begin this discussion of mutual respect.

The video, *A Choice for K'aila,* which documents K'aila's parents' choice and the court's decision,[7] brings many of the aspects of the theme of mutual respect to the foreground: first and foremost, respect for persons, but also respect for different kinds of knowledge and for differing cultural and religious values. Within this intense, heart-breaking story, the people who are involved are K'aila (the baby), his mother, his father, the doctor(s), hospital personnel, friends and other family members, and medical, legal, and social welfare experts. Agencies and institutions such as the social welfare system, the justice system, and the medical system are also in need of careful consideration. It becomes clear that different kinds of knowledge were considered in the ethical and legal decision making that surrounded K'aila's short life: medical, native, spiritual, community, parental, cognitive, intuitive, emotional, and physical. Inherent in this assembly of persons, agencies, institutions, and kinds of knowledge are differences in power and authority.

GATHERING AROUND K'AILA

In the video *A Choice for K'aila: May Parents Refuse a Transplant for Their Child?* K'aila's parents describe the experience of saying "no" to a liver transplant for their infant son who was found to have terminal liver disease.[8] The video follows the path of K'aila's diagnosis of liver disease to the point where this parents take him to an adjacent province because they fear that their child will be taken into custody by local Social Services authorities. The video also explores the physician's decision to refer the family to Social Services when they do not accept his advice to proceed with liver transplantation assessment for K'aila. The parents discuss how they came to make the choice for their son and how they had to defend that choice in a court of law. The final decision by the Provincial Court of Saskatchewan supported the parents and dismissed the application of the Minister of Social Services for temporary care of K'aila. At 11 months of age, K'aila died at home in the arms of his family.

In the drama, which portrays K'aila's life and death, two approaches to decision making are used and could be seen as colliding. One approach, the four-principle approach, based on the ethical principles of autonomy, beneficence, non-maleficence, and justice, is juxtaposed to an approach that Lesley Paulette, K'aila's mother, calls the whole-person model.

The four-principle approach is based on cognitive rational analysis and the application of principles to the situational dilemma, with little attention to emotion.[9] In the whole-person model, attention is focussed on four levels of understanding that are intimately involved in the parents' decision making for K'aila: mind/reason, body/action, spirit/vision, and heart/feeling (see figure 1).[10] The whole-person model does not reject the rational, cognitive understanding (of the transplantation, the disease process, the drug needs, and so on); rather, it integrates factual medical knowledge (mind and reason) with personal knowledge (feeling and vision), which Lesley Paulette said was "already available to me in spirit and in heart."[11] Factual knowledge is understood as *one* source of knowledge among several.

The Whole-Person Model

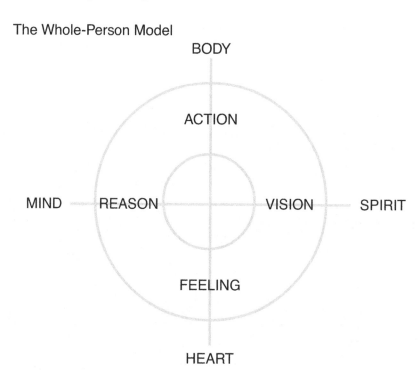

Figure 1. From Lesley Paulette, "A Choice for K'aila," *Humane Medicine* 9, no. 1 (1993): 13-7, p. 14. © 1993, Multimed. Used with permission.

The pediatrician, in discussing his decision to refer K'aila
to the provincial Department of Social Services for protection
and treatment, states that he wanted to give the infant a chance
to live long enough to make decisions about his own treatments. Appealing to the principles of beneficence and non-
maleficence, the pediatrician felt it was his duty to give K'aila
a chance at life. Here transplantation (and the possibility of
life) is thought to be beneficial, whereas no transplantation
(and the reality of death) is the ultimate harm. As K'aila's physician, the pediatrician became, by default, the one who made
choices for a community of pediatricians and for the public at
large. Out of consideration for K'aila's life, K'aila's parents,
and for the community at large, the physician decided that
wider discussion of the choices must occur. He said that he
could not make this decision by himself and neither could
the parents. The doctor knew that any decisions made in
K'aila's situation would affect decisions made in the future in
similar situations. He may have been concerned, too, that if
K'aila's parents were not completely sure about their decision
to forego treatment that they might have misgivings in the
future. By broadening the community of decision makers to
include the courts, such doubts may have been less likely to
occur.

In the end, the decision that K'aila's parents wanted for
him was upheld by the courts. In the final decision, the court
stated that the parents had made a decision based not only on
the medical facts, but had "given a much more profound consideration to other components."[12] The story of K'aila and the
subsequent court decision show regard for various kinds of
knowledge—medical (body), rationality (mind), love and feeling (heart), and the interconnection of all life (spirit).

While the whole-person model and the four-principle approach of ethical decision making seem to collide in this situation, perhaps the primary difficulty is different. The relationship between the parents and the physician became confrontational, with the doctor *threatening* to report the family
to Social Services and the parents *escaping* to another jurisdiction in fear that their child would be apprehended. Was
mutual respect experienced in the situation with K'aila? It
seems not. The parents did not feel respected by the physi-

cian in their choice of palliative rather than aggressive care for their child. The physician did not feel respected when the parents took their child out of his care and fled to another location and another physician. How could it have been different? Both the parents and the physician wanted to make a decision that was best for the child, but they did not respect the other's point of view. On the one side, the physician could not understand the parents' refusal to offer their child a treatment that, in his mind, would give the child a good chance at life. The parents, on the other side, could not understand that aggressive treatment, which would cause their son intense suffering and life-long medical supervision, was the best (and, indeed, only) solution to the tragedy of life-threatening liver disease.

Although referring difficult healthcare decisions to the court has occurred in a number of situations,[13] there are other options, such as consultation with an ethics committee. More importantly, removing the threat of apprehension in order to maintain conversations between parents, physicians, other healthcare givers, and family members might have preserved the relational aspects of this situation. An attitude of mutual respect might have mitigated the power of the physician and the vulnerability of the parents, and may have allowed a less confrontational approach. It may be necessary for us to consider a completely different approach, an approach that places in question the notion that the child is, or should be, the ultimate decision maker.

Both the whole-person and the four-principle approach are based on the theory that the child is, or should be, the decision maker. In both models, K'aila is seen as a separate, autonomous individual who *should* be able to make the decision for himself. It is his immaturity that leaves him dependent, powerless, and, indeed, choice-less. The parents and the physician, and even the legal system, became proxy decision makers[14] for the infant, because K'aila, the proper and only one to make the choice, was not capable of independent decision making; someone else had to make the decision for him. Immediately, we encounter questions: At what age would he be capable of making a fully independent choice about transplantation? How could mutual respect (the nucleus of relationship) help to uncover the issues at stake? How can a relational perspective change our understanding of making choices to one that is shared, rather than autonomous, one that connects people, rather than separates them from each other? We present a relational notion of personhood, that of fostering autonomy, which accommodates the immaturity of K'aila without negating his personhood. Fostering autonomy is not dependent upon age, cognitive abilities, or other factors.

PERSONHOOD

Think again about K'aila. K'aila was not alone. He was born into the arms of a family: his mother, Lesley, his father, François, and his brother, Thaidene. They were all present at his birth. At 11 months of age K'aila died. Again, he was within the arms of his family, with his mother and father talking and singing to him, to make his death as tranquil and peaceful as possible. They did not want K'aila to be afraid. As K'aila died, his mother said that her "heart broke wide open,"[15] and she experienced a love and sense of inner peace that she had not known before. The decision about what she needed to do for K'aila came one night in the hospital, when the baby could not settle and had an intravenous line in his tiny foot. She took him out of his crib and brought him into her narrow cot.

As he snuggled into my arms and began to nurse, he relaxed and fell asleep. I watched him sleeping peacefully, and it became clear to me what I had to do for him. I imagined him like a butterfly, so beautiful, indeed exquisite, and yet so fragile. With my palm open wide, he had lighted on my hand and now rested there a few moments, his wings shimmering in the light. I longed for him to stay forever, but I knew that at any time he might flutter his wings and be gone. The only way I could hang on to him would be to close my hand around him, to entrap him in my grasp. However, I knew that in doing so I would run the real risk of harming him; I might open my fingers again to find his wings broken and crippled, his colours faded and smudged. I knew in that moment I must keep my palm open and let him take flight when the time came. . . . We [my husband

and I] struggled and questioned it together until we came to a common conviction. We prayed and meditated for weeks, even months, until we reached a place where we felt whole and at peace with our decision.[16]

K'aila's life and death speak of the connection of persons. This connection, this interconnection, is so readily seen in the beginning of life—with babies and young children. K'aila did, and could, not live or die without connection to his parents or someone taking the parental role. We can easily agree that all children deserve such a connection—to parents or someone else close and committed to them. All people need connections with others, for it is in the centrality of relationships that the self is constituted.

In looking more closely at K'aila's life, we see a relational sense of personhood showing through. Lesley Paulette talks of her experience of decision making with K'aila, because "of all the people who knew K'aila," she says, "I knew him best. I had spent the most time in contact with him, and was in the best position to communicate with him about what he wanted."[17]John Macmurray contemplates the meaning of communication between mother and son and says, "the impulse to communication is his [the human infant's] sole adaptation to the world into which he is born. Implicit and unconscious as it may be, yet it is sufficient to constitute the mother-child relation as the basic form of human existence, as a personal mutuality, as a 'You and I' with a common life."[18]Macmurray develops his notion of the *person* further:

> Thus human experience is, in principle, shared experience; human life, even in its most individual elements, is a common life; and human behaviour carries always, in its inherent structure, a reference to the personal Other. All this may be summed up by saying that the unit of personal existence is not the individual, but two persons in personal relation; and that we are persons not by individual right, but in virtue of our relation to one another. The personal is constituted by personal relatedness. The unit of the personal is not the "I," but the "You and I." [19]

Macmurray speaks to the ebb and flow of human personhood—the relational interdependent reality of being a person. Emmanuel Lévinas also challenges the "solitude of Being," and proposes that we be governed by "one's infinite obligation to the other person"[20] brought most vividly to our attention by the face of another.

K'aila's mother says, "I tried as often as I could just to be quiet and to listen to him tell me what he wanted . . . in the quiet moments with K'aila I felt most lucid . . . it became clear to me what I had to do for him."[21] The personhood of both K'aila and his mother was a "You and I" connection. K'aila was not able to be completely autonomous, but his mother, by her attention, listening, observing, touching, began to know what he wanted; she fostered his autonomy with her closeness—being *with* him so she could be *for* him.[22] Lesley Paulette would not be able make a decision for K'aila in the way she did without first being with him, listening to him, loving him. The doctor could not be with K'aila in the way his mother was—unless he too had attempted to be that close to him. When one thinks of personhood in this relational way, one can wonder if it is ever possible to make absolutely autonomous decisions, especially weighty decisions of life and death.

The pediatrician, in wanting to have K'aila live until he could make life and death decisions for himself, may not accept Macmurray's definition of person as the "You and I." The principle of autonomy, the "I," in striving for independence and self-determination free from influences of others, is paramount and well-developed in current Western ethical thought. Although it is not necessarily held by many cultures, [23] those who hold the principle of respect for autonomy as primary would not accept the notion that parents and their children are intimately connected morally, that both are constituted by the "You and I," not just the "I." Yet Macmurray takes his argument further. He says that the person, as the "You and I," is not a reality only during infancy, but for all of human life. The goal of maturity, in this articulation of the person, is not independence, but *interdependence*: "If the *terminus a quo* of the personal life is a helpless total dependence on the Other, the *terminus ad quem* is not independence, but a mutual interdependence of equals."[24] An independent notion of person, as an independent "I," would have K'aila live until he had the ability to make a decision for himself. An interdependent notion of person, as a "You and I," would take the whole family relationship, as well as the physician into context, and for some families and their physicians the decision might be different. In any case, if K'aila had lived by having the transplantation, he would still never have to make the decision his parents were required to make with him.

In an interdependent notion of personhood, as a child moves toward maturity and independence, he or she would still be interdependent. Or, as an adult who moves toward the end of life moves toward dependency and loss of ability, he or she would still be interdependent. If this notion of person is correct, then the unit of the person is the interdependent "You and I," and neither the independent nor dependent "I." In this sense, K'aila's parents made a choice *with* K'aila. As R. Melvin Keiser notes, for many people important decisions are never "individualistic . . . [for] without companions, collaborators, teachers, corroborating witnesses, I am at the mercy of my imaginations. . . . In conversations, literal and metaphoric, we clarify and corroborate our choices in their depths, breadth, discernment of the divine, and religious foundation."[25] Choice is made *with* K'aila, not *for* him. Similar decision making occurs at the other end of life, with family, often children, making decisions they feel are most closely aligned with the choices the elder person or parent would have wanted. Care must be taken to see that personhood always attends to the needs of the other as well as the self. Having only a self-interested focus would lead to harm.

The notion of the person as a rational, self-motivated, and self-aware human being is challenged by the experience of dementia and the intuitions felt by the people who care for those with dementia. Christine Harrison proposes a broader notion of person that might be more useful in understanding obligations to individuals with dementia: a *narrative* view (a person as subject of a unified life) or a *gestalt* view (a person with changing entities that are parts of a whole being who has character, function, and role).[26] Could it be that, even at the

end of life, when people can no longer make decisions by or
for themselves (in matters of competency), that one could make
decisions *with* the person rather than *for* the person? A choice
is made *with* one's senile mother, not *for* her. Both the parents
and the children here are involved in the personhood of their
children and parents. Yet, from this view, even fully competent adults are interdependent.

INTERDEPENDENCE

In the 1960s, philosophers such as John Macmurray[27] and
H. Richard Niebuhr[28] wrote about persons as relational beings
and that responsiveness to self and responsiveness to others
are necessary components of ethics; yet it was years before
philosophers (stimulated by feminist philosophy) and healthcare professionals (especially those working in chronic care)[29]
began to raise questions about the emphasis—indeed, the overemphasis—on autonomy as a primary and overriding principle, and the impossibility of completely autonomous choices.
Why these early works (for example, those of Macmurray and
Niebuhr) have been ignored by the mainstream Western philosophical community, which understands persons as "robustly
individualistic,"[30] is a question worthy of further study.

More recently, particularly since the research of Carol
Gilligan in 1983, feminist scholars have contested the received
definition of personhood as disembodied, rational, autonomous, separate, isolated, and abstract, as in the term "generalized other."[31] As Seyla Benhabib notes, an individual "wholly
constituted by the possession of moral rights, based on the
capacity for rationally autonomous moral agency or by self-
consciousness [is an] exceedingly thin"[32] notion of what it
means to be a person. This thin, bare-bones, standard account
of personhood leads to a thin, bare-bones, arms-length notion
of respect for others as separated and distanced "rights-bear-
ers." This notion of personhood cannot acknowledge the
shapes and circumstances of individual human lives, does
not engage one emotionally, leads to oppositional, combative
conceptions of tolerance, and tends to foster victimization,
says Robin Dillon.[33] She adds that respect "recognizes us si-

multaneously as separate and self-synthesizing and as embedded in innumerable networks of personal, social, and institutional relationships with others in ways that mark our very being as relational and interdependent."[34] A person, as an interdependent being, is both separate from others (independent) and connected to others (dependent) at the same time; that is an enlarged view of what it means to be a person.

Of course, to be interdependent and relational does *not* release one from self-determinacy and autonomy; yet, within interdependency, autonomy is active and changing, rather than achieved or not achieved. With interdependency, one still can be alone, and mutual respectfulness recognizes this aloneness and forbids any attempt, even for the other person's sake, to rob anyone of independence. Responsibility for the other person never consists of assuming responsibility for that which belongs to, or can be practiced by, that person.[35] The notion of interdependency with its attention to respect—a mutual and developing respect—protects against paternalism; yet one must always be attentive to paternalism's seductive rationality that can lead one to think, "I know best!" Anne Donchin reminds us that a self is "shaped by both social experience and individual choice,"[36] and, within the particular vulnerability of that patient's experience, whether he or she is child, adult, elderly, or demented, there is need for caregivers to actively nurture and foster capacities for the patient's continuing human flourishing. A relational personhood, an interdependent personhood, fosters, rather than assumes, autonomy. Respectful attention to existential aloneness involves closeness as well as distance.

Robert Burt, a lawyer, suggests that professionals, lawyers, and even the judges/courts should not take on the job of deciding *for* someone (a role that is now expected of judges and courts).[37] Rather, Burt says, the role of healthcare professionals, lawyers, and judges is to facilitate continued conversation between doctors and patients, careproviders and the recipients of care, to ensure debate and continued conversation over time. The discussion may never be conclusively ended, but only soothed, muted, and attenuated, because the question of separate or fused self-boundaries is never conclusively answered in any interpersonal relation. Burt, in conversation with Dax Cowart, a severely burned man who endured years of painful treatments despite his requests to be allowed to die, says that we "define one another for one another [as we are not] isolated creatures, popped into this world, who chart ourselves only by what's in our head. We are intensely social creatures."[38] So, "If you die, I lose too. We are in this together." We are not really completely separate beings; we are connected in strong social ways. Decisions, especially healthcare decisions, need to be negotiated between people, *with* each other, doctors and patients, husbands and wives, parents and children and/or friends, in order to understand shared meanings about what should be done. In these kinds of partnerships, all persons, as moral agents, are free to accept and decline the interpretation that each offers, until they reach a meaning that both affirm.[39] We are alone on our personal journey, because each person experiences life in an individual manner. At the same time, though, everybody encounters many common situations. We cannot walk in the other person's shoes, but, just by walking in shoes ourselves, we can partially understand the experiences of others as we, too, have similar experiences. To gain understanding we can walk beside others and talk with them. It means that we need to talk together about serious issues. What does my life mean to me? What kinds of values do we hold? What kind of care and treatment do we want at the end of life? These are difficult things to talk about.

The strengths and demands of an articulation of the person as both individualistic and relational are complex. Within a relational notion of personhood, one is committed to both self (as person) and other (as person) at the same time, with the obligation to support independent action whenever possible. Attention, within a relational definition of personhood, is directed to both *responsibility for* and *responsiveness in* relations,[40] and to be *for* another person in order to be *with* the person.[41] This notion differs from John Stuart Mill's division of acts into those that are either self-regarding (as an egoistic person, living life only for the self) and those that are other-regarding (altruistic, living life only for others) in nature. Mill's view is an either/or situation rather that both/and. Dax Cowart agrees with Mill that "when an act is self-regarding in nature, the individual should be left to make his or her own decisions."[42] In healthcare practice, however, when there is interest in fostering autonomy and when coming to a decision is a shared experience, the caregiver must stay involved and spend time with the person, time that is respectful and extensive. "The commitment is enormously burdensome for the caretaker to take on these situations. But that to me," says Burt, "is the heart of caretaking."[43] Could it be that the *full* meaning of respect is this concept of *mutuality*? In mutuality we need to be present with the other with both heart and mind. It is not easy to practice the value of mutual respect in day-to-day life.

The notion of mutual respect sustains and integrates both self-interest (the self-respectful moral subject) and other-interested (the respectful moral agent) in one person. Yet how can a person be both self-interested and other-interested at the same time without jeopardizing either or being in continual conflict? In the next section, we focus on the attentiveness, the relational space of unconditional regard, needed for mutual respect to occur—attention to the self, attention to the other, and the connection between self and other.

RELATIONAL RESPECT

To respect something one must focus on it. As Robin Dillon notes, "We respect something by paying careful attention to it and taking it seriously. To ignore, neglect, or disregard something, or to dismiss it lightly, thoughtlessly, or carelessly is to not respect it."[44] This is true also with people: Persons need attention as unique beings with varying values, culture, race, gender, attitudes, experiences, and desires. Attention to questions like *Who am I? Who are You?* and *What is our connection?* are among the first to be asked in a relational ethic.[45]

RESPECT FOR SELF

Mutual respect begins with self-respect. Mutual respect is *person*-focused, and, as Dillon notes, "its vision encompasses oneself equally with others."[46] It is self-awareness, not self-absorption, that we are discussing. While self-respect is not "belly button gazing" we may often think about others, "Don't be so egocentric, don't worry about yourself." We cannot have a relational ethic—a relation with clients where we look at their issues and their particulars—without looking at our own. If mutual respect (or, as Dillon terms it, "care respect") "regards all persons as equally valuable, equally worthy of care and of protection from harm, it cannot countenance sacrificing the well-being of one for the sake of another."[47] This means, of course, that mutual respect expects one to care for oneself, and caring for oneself includes continually growing in self-understanding. Caring for the self as an "I" develops with the developing personhood, the "You and I."

People grow and change throughout life. Yet is the question *Who am I?* truly a question for ethics? Can the ancient and perennial commandment to "Know thyself" be a moral responsibility for healthcare practitioners? If we say that understanding oneself is a concern of ethics, we will also have to say that discovering what is right or wrong for oneself is an individual responsibility, for, according to Keiser, "only individuals can discover what decision is appropriate to their commitments."[48](This does not mean that there are no legal rights that members of a society agree to respect.) As we know more about ourselves, we begin to see more clearly how we respond to others, what our values are, what dismays us, what engages us, and how we can grow and change in our response.

The question of *self-knowledge* is the raising of consciousness of our tacit commitments and prejudices, a matter of moral consciousness. The question *Who am I?* is a question of humility, of self in relation to others—not in a self-effacing way, but in a self-understanding way. This attitude of humility is not a virtue that can be cultivated by oneself, but is a relational, inquisitive openness to find out more about our own values, beliefs, and sense of rightness.[49] We learn moral consciousness through education and custom.[50]We come to know ourselves through relations with others: just as a child comes to know him- or herself from interaction with the mother or father; just as a woman comes to know herself as a mother through interaction with her child; or just as a person comes to know the self as a nurse or doctor through interaction with patients and each other. So we can see that the question *Who am I?* as a healthcare practitioner—who supports another person, who nourishes the other to grow and heal, or who fosters the well-being of others—*can* be a first question of ethics.

Who am I as a midwife, as a physician, as a lawyer? *Who am I* as a parent or as a friend? *Who am I* as a patient? What are my competencies? What are my values? What, above all, do I cherish? What is my passion, my *daimon*?[51] Do I cherish the notion of the sanctity of life at all costs, or is freedom from intractable pain more important to me than life itself? How am I, as a nurse or doctor, different from other nurses or doctors? Have I lost my individuality in taking on a role? These questions lead to increased self-awareness and self-understanding, which help a person reflect on what makes him or her different from others and unique. As Jon Amundson and colleagues note, often the self-learning of practitioners in healthcare situations is painful and lifelong, gained through "bumping into their own rigidities, bruising themselves, or stumbling over their clients," which means that we develop "an openness to ourselves and what we possess as naive or unique resources, but also to accepting the same in others."[52] Learning about ourselves is a joint venture.

Healthcare practitioners, whether they are personal care attendants, physicians, or rehabilitation therapists, have expertise that deserves recognition and respect. Relational ethics requires competency and knowledge; competency in skills, theory and knowledge, and ability are vitally important. The expertise of the pediatrician in *A Choice for K'aila* is not placed in question in the exploration of this scenario. Rather, his expertise is highly prized. If there were a question to be asked, it would be the question of certainty—the conviction that his approach to care was the right and the only one. As Amundson and colleagues state, one of the temptations of certainty is the loss of self-questioning: "Expertise . . . may silence not only our clients but ourselves as therapists."[53] Silencing of questioning leads to ethical harm through the loss of consideration of alternative views and understandings and the subordination of some kinds of knowledge (such as indigenous or

local knowledge) and experience (moment-by-moment living
in the situation) to expertise. Respect for and knowledge of
oneself, as well as acknowledgment of the diverse perspectives from our human complexity, means that healthcare is
like a journey, not one with a specified destination, but one
that is involved in "a continual process of departure, not only
for our clients but for ourselves," according to Amundson and
colleagues.[54]

RESPECT FOR OTHERS

We started this section by saying that mutual respect begins with self-respect. We can now also say that mutual respect begins with respect for others. Self-respect and respect
for others are respect *for persons,* and do not occur in a linear
fashion. Self-respect and respect for others have been or can
be learned, at the same time. One cannot truly respect others
without a deep respect for oneself; one cannot truly respect
oneself without a deep respect for others.

In healthcare, the interest in mutual respect addresses both
Who is the person as caregiver? and *Who is the person as
patient or client?* How does one know the other? What competencies (and this means more than just mental capacity)
does one have? What values and beliefs? What desires, wishes,
plans, hopes, and so forth? What difference does it make
whether a person is addressed as Alice, Mrs. Brown, Dr. Johns,
or Ralph Mitchell? One physician, Oscar London, tells of losing a patient because the receptionist called an elderly patient "Rose" instead of "Mrs. Schwartz." London says, too,
that he has "to stifle an impulse to call patients, especially
young ones, by their first names . . . [but respect] demands
that the doctor offer to let Mrs. Rose Schwartz call him by *his*
first name if he wants to address Mrs. Schwartz by *her* first
name."[55] Calling each other by name gives personal recognition, confirms support, and affirms humanness. Yet there is
need for caution. As Carole Ann Taylor notes, "Any narrative
that reveals a privileged frame of reference . . . necessitates a
difficult revisioning of relationality (how I stand in relation
to Others)."[56] If we take liberties in naming, as in calling another by name in a superficial way, it can lead to more alien-

ation, like "taking one's name in vain." It is appropriate to ask a person how they wish to be addressed: "What name do you prefer?"—so that naming each other supports relationship rather than ruptures it.

Yet is naming really an ethical concern? Sometimes patients are labelled difficult, manipulating, deceitful, cunning, strong-willed, compulsive, envious, greedy, selfish, or narcissistic. These words were used to describe a young woman with anorexia nervosa who did not respond to treatment in a case related by Philip C. Hébert and Michael A. Weingarten.[57] Sometimes when patients ask or respond in ways that caregivers disagree with, they may be referred to as being "out to lunch," noncompliant, or difficult. Would we use these descriptors for people who are cooperative with treatment plans? What does such labelling do to a person? Perhaps it is the difficult patients, says Joan Liaschenko, who need most respect: "It's those hard ones that really need a conscious effort at respect, a conscious effort of taking the time, a conscious effort to figure out how—if you can make a connection with them, how you can do it. And sometimes you can't."[58] Perhaps we have responsibility to *go out to lunch* with those who are "out to lunch"—that is, to strive to make connections however we can.

"There can be no reaching out into the realm of the incommunicable . . . unless the physician becomes a fellow traveller, a fellow explorer," says Oliver Sacks, the famous neurologist and author of *Awakening*.[59] He says that doctor and patient, together, must create languages that bridge the gulf between them. The ethical question *Who are You?* is not merely used to find out the medical or social history, or to obtain a detailed account of the signs and symptoms (all of which are important), but to explore the ways and means of how "You and I" can make connections with each other as persons. Because we need to recognize the power inherent in the right to initiate naming, we believe that this example is ethical in nature, rather than merely etiquette.

However much we are similar, we are also ultimately different. Taking our differences seriously might be another first step in mutual respect. We began this discussion of mutual respect by describing the different disciplines, different genders, different power bases, and different kinds of knowledge that are present in any healthcare situation, whether in our research group or in institutions or agencies, whether it is with K'aila's parents, or K'aila's doctor. Nurses and physicians see the same situation from different perspectives; sometimes nurses focus on a person's experience of the illness (the whole person), and physicians focus on the problem of the illness (the disease process)—and sometimes it is the other way around. How can respect for both *foci* be equally valued as important in the care of the patient? How can respect for all persons, nurse and doctor and patient, who live in these roles, be mutually encouraged? Respect for difference, whether in roles, gender, knowledge, or disease (acknowledging the current hierarchy of diseases—for example, heart disease is often experienced as more "acceptable" than AIDS) can only be experienced as respect for the person who lives the gender, the role, the knowledge, or the disease.

Mutual respect in healthcare means respecting and valuing diversity. As Annette Brown notes, mutual respect means "unconditional acceptance, recognition, and acknowledgment"[60] of all persons, without attempting to make everyone the same or treating everyone as if they are the same. People who respect each other in relationship continually help us all to confront prejudices, ignorances, misunderstanding, and negative attitudes—about ourselves and about others. It is only through encounters with others that we can understand the complex ways in which culture, race, class, and identities find expression in our lives.[61] Of course, even uniqueness can be taken too far. If someone is absolutely different, there is no point of contact, and, thus, no possibility of relationship. The holocaust in Nazi Germany demonstrates the extent of destruction and violence that happens when difference (ethnic, religious, or ableness) is taken to the point where there is a complete loss of relationship. We need to know how we are the same, not just how we are different. Joan Liaschenko notes, "When we attempt to bridge the gap between self and other, we share in a moral history by acknowledging the commonalties of need we all share."[62] Bridging the gap is done through focus on relationship, the *and*, that connects us to each other.

THE CONNECTION: THE *AND*

Mutual respect involves the *and*—the way respect for person (as "You and I") is enacted. In healthcare situations the *and* is experienced through conversation or dialogue—a back and forth exchange. Responsiveness includes interpretation not ruled by passion or principles, but, as Neibuhr says, "interpretation of events as intelligible, rational events in the determined whole"[63]—best found in responding to the questions *What is going on?* and *What is the fitting thing to do?*

In general practice, though, instead of conversation, the medical interview (or history taking) is a common tool of one-way information gathering. An extreme example is told by a person who is interviewed by 12 different caregivers, each charting with a check list. In spite of these many interviews, the patient felt he had yet to tell his story the way he wanted. Yet even the word *interview* can bring us back to the significance of the relation.[64] The original meaning of the word interview, from *entrevu*, means "to see each other."[65] Seeing each other suggests the opportunity of seeing the views of each other, sharing different viewpoints, partaking of an inter-view. Inter-view, as conversation, needs to explore beliefs about an illness, disease, even life itself. Although we may perceive some beliefs as better than others, all beliefs and attitudes are legitimate and need to be expressed and shared. In modern life, we tend to look for final answers, answers that are certain and reliable, and definite solutions to problems; caregivers want to provide this kind of care, and patients and clients have come to expect it. Yet Dianne Tapp discusses the need to accept the legitimacy of different points of view. Through acceptance rather than judgment (to label, blame, or invalidate), we respect both the expertise and experience of family members and professionals.[66] Mutual respect means that there is a need to accept the legitimacy of different points of view, and, by accepting the legitimacy of other points of view, creating space for mutual respect to occur. There is, of course, the need to offer views that are thought to be most appropriate, based on the scientific reasoning, but this must be done in a way that does not negate others' beliefs and knowledge, which may differ from the dominant view. Tapp talks of "offering ideas *as invitations* to reflection,"[67] when people can listen, question, and clarify a response that is best for them. In order to move from "interview" to "inter-view," from information-giving to conversation, there needs to be an openness to respecting and to appreciating different points of view. The concern of the caregiver to do things in the other person's best interests has often been expressed as the need to convince the person to take a particular action or comply with specific knowledge and advice. Rather, we suggest, it is better for caregivers to ask questions and offer ideas that may enable patients and their families to entertain more effective possibilities for addressing the problems and dilemmas they may encounter.[68]

In an inter-view, the healthcare practitioner is also asked to be self-questioning and open to new possibilities of understanding. The reciprocity of such an approach means that vulnerability or humility, as well as confidence and expertise, are inherent in dialogue. In conversation we respond in an appropriate manner to what is said to us. "Suitable responses are multiple, not just one," as R. Melvin Keiser notes.[69] In dialogue, it is not just ideas or concepts that are present; rather, in dialogue much more occurs in the total meaning of the moment, such as the emphasis given, the flow of the ideas, clear or ambiguous worlds that are chosen, the rhythms, and the sounds.[70] Within a relational ethic perspective, caregivers are not only concerned with understanding you as a disease or health problem, but you as a whole person that connects with me as a whole person, even for a short time—during this procedure, this chemotherapy treatment, or this bath—so that we may explore, together, how to involve you in making your own decisions about what kinds of treatment you want when you are ill or how you want to be treated when you are dying.[71] It may even have to do with learning more about ourselves (me learning about me and you learning more about you)—about values, about beliefs, or about what we want in life. In an environment where everyone (patients, family, colleagues) wants definitive answers, cures, or problems solved, attention to the whole person (both self and other) and to relationship as a journey is not easy. Healthcare professionals deal with this all the time, this back and forth thing of people we're caring for, and see the pain, stay in the pain, and are totally aware of the other as a full person. We do this by *being with* patients. Being with patients in this way makes us vulnerable.

Although goals are important in healthcare, what often gets lost is how the goals are enacted. To the mother of K'aila, the goal was safe passage of her child, even if he did not live; to the doctor of K'aila, the goal was survival of the child. Goals fit nicely into the teleological (having to do with ends) or deontological (having to do with duties) theories of healthcare ethics, such as *What is my goal, ideal, or telos?* or *What is the law?* or *What is my duty?* The relational approach, which Niebuhr calls "responsibility,"[72] might react more directly to the questions *What is going on in the life of the child; the family? What is the fitting thing to do in this situation?* In the end, it may be necessary for the parents and the physician to consult the wider community (for example, an ethics committee, a council, or the court). But following the lead of Robert Burt, the work of the ethics committee, and the court, is to keep the conversation between all parties ongoing, and not to identify anyone—child, parents, physician, or judge—"as ultimate and exclusive decision-maker [which] aborts the very process of communal collaboration by which each of us sustains individual identity."[73] Identifying *the* choice maker, even at the level of the court, relieves individuals of the distress of making these hard choices and leaves people to turn away from each other rather than "toward each other for mutual support and recognition."[74] Identifying *the* choice maker makes it possible, and indeed may make it necessary, for healthcare practitioners to "wash their hands" and refer the case to the legal jurisdiction, and it makes it possible, and indeed may make it necessary, for parents to pick up their child and flee.

According to Leonard Angel, relational ethics holds that "the key to living well lies in disentangling and understanding the multiplicity of our roles."[75] Roles define connections between people in healthcare; in fact, roles define relationships. Roles are not masks or costumes that people put on, but are ways of being—ways of living life. What does it mean to be a nurse, a doctor, a father, or a mother? Is the person the same person in a different role? Does there need to be congruence of person in different roles? When a role is understood as *a way of being*, relationships are involved. As soon as one takes on the role of parent, moral responsibilities to the child are present. If one is a nurse, there is a patient. If one is a gerontologist, there is an elder. If one is a midwife, there is a pregnant laboring woman. The role defines responsibility and relationship.

Some terms have become so general and/or technical that the roles and their relationships are lost. Think of the common term, *significant other*, as a term that could mean lover, legal wife or husband, common-law spouse, child, or close friend. Yet *significant other* misses the moral commitment that the word lover, child, wife, or husband identify. More startling are technical terms, like *intact survivor*, used by professionals to mean a seriously ill newborn who has recovered well enough so there is a good chance of living without disability. In everyday language, *intact survivor* is a "healthy baby." *Intact survivor* is a technical term, but "healthy baby" is both a social and moral term. The term "healthy baby" carries with it the social connection to a mother, a father, a family, a community, and it carries moral implications—a baby needs care, needs a loving person committed to its growth and development. When we say the words "a healthy baby," we anticipate moral commitment; whereas, when we use *an intact survivor,* our language loses any connection with parent, needs, or commitment. Even in using the term *young offender*, we can easily forget that we are talking about a child or an adolescent, and our focus shifts to the *offense*. Of course, these technical terms are value-laden, useful in their objectivity and scientific clarity. Yet relationships can be lost in the use of technical terms, whereas, with role-related terms, such as nurse or doctor, the commitment between the self, as nurse or doctor, and other, as patient, is implicitly present.

It is possible, of course, that one can also hide behind roles. When social and cultural rankings and status, especially, are attributed to roles, relationships may be limited and destroyed. One way to hide behind roles is through a uniform—the white coat, the stethoscope, the dark suit and tie, and so on. Another way is the use of names: titles for some, first names for

others. On the one hand, being a healthcare professional offers people the opportunity to take on caring roles, which provide the possibility to interact with people in important and
life-changing ways. On the other hand, the dangers of self-
interested people who take on caregiving roles, such as parents who hurt children, doctors who abuse patients, nurses
who manipulate or coerce vulnerable clients, children who
rob elderly parents, need to be addressed. Such abuses demonstrate the moral nature of these roles.

One major concern with mutual respect is power. There
has been considerable questioning about different notions of
power: power over, power with, or to empower. The focus on
power also brings attention to powerlessness, both of patients
and of professionals. In the next section, we will explore power
in the relational ethic of mutual respect, which may effec-
tively turn power on its head and put it in its proper place.

MUTUAL POWER

Mutual respect mitigates power's potential to damage. Mutual respect puts power in the proper place, with each person
able to live within his or her own position of power. Robin
Dillon says, "respect requires not so much refraining from interference as recognizing our power to make and unmake each
other as persons and exercising this power wisely and carefully."[76] How is power used in healthcare practice to dimin-
ish the ability of persons, both as caregivers and patients, to
live out their own power? How can mutual respect encourage
wise and appropriate use of power? Can power be seen as
shared rather than dominating? Can the feeling of powerlessness, especially in the face of suffering and death, be understood in an attitude of respect to the person and for life itself?
How do scientific, abstract discourses hide issues of power?

The midwifery relation is one where respect for choices
of the pregnant, laboring, and mothering woman are paramount.[77] Yet there are moments when the midwife can say to
the laboring woman, "Do this, now!" At that moment the midwife exerts her power, a power based on knowledge and expertise that must, at a particular moment, be respected with-

out hesitancy or conversation—for the health of both mother and baby. Such expression of power is not seen as power of the expert over the naïve or powerless, but power granted through mutual respect. The laboring woman hears the urgency in the midwife's tone and responds to the command as an appropriate and valued expression of power. This is not a time for the woman to exert her own preference or choice. Appropriate power, here, is relational power.

Frequently we hear of patients who do not want to make decisions for themselves or do not want to know too much about the details of the medical problem they are experiencing. Does this mean that they give over their power to the healthcare practitioner? Or does it signal a need for greater attention by the caregiver to find ways to assist the patient and family to gain confidence in their own abilities to understand and share the power, as they are able? Could it mean that people are afraid of the abandonment so easily experienced when decision making is not shared, and when individuals are given arm's-length respect?

Perhaps the way to put power in its place is to focus on the power in the relation rather than power *over* (over-power) or even power *given* (em-power). When considering power in relation to mutual respect, perhaps we need to attend to power *between* or *with* (giving place for power). Power *between* recognizes power differences, it holds power within view, faces power directly, or, in the words of Humberto Maturana and Francisco Varela, holds power in an attitude of permanent vigilance.[78] Perhaps relational ethics gives attention and space to *re*-power—to consider ways to remind persons of the power that rightfully belongs within each of us as human persons. The notion of fostering autonomy is really fostering relational power, fostering space for persons to find and take hold of the personal inner power that is already present. It may also require a fostering of outer power to assist each other to enact one's own inner power.

Power is often related to the notion of independence and control found within the principle of autonomy and authority. However, when dependence is seen as a significant aspect of humanness and not a failure of individuation or maturity, power can be shared rather than be hierarchical. As Gilligan notes, "Being dependent, then, no longer means being helpless, powerless, and without control; rather, it signifies a conviction that one is able to have an effect on others. One is interdependent."[79] Dependence, within an interdependent world, recognizes that both self and other have power, not at each other's expense, but in order to build community and to promote dignity and self-worth. Activities such as listening, willingness to help, taking time to understand, and being present for another take on moral dimensions that keep power in view.

When people are not listened to, or when they cannot voice their own questions and values, there is a sense of powerlessness. The ethical concern about *informed consent* is seen as one of the major ways to keep the power where it belongs, within each person, within both caregiver and patient. As Mark Kuczewski says, within the concept of informed consent, "the person is conceptualized as possessing a sphere of protected activity or privacy free from unwanted interference. Within this zone of privacy, one is able to exercise his or her liberty and discretion. Within this protected sphere take place disclosure, comprehension, and choice, which express the patient's right of self-determination over her body."[80] In the current definition of informed consent, the family (as defined by the patient) is not part of the decision-making team, especially if the patient is able (cognitively able) to make her or his own decisions. In fact, there is rightful concern about the family's possibly competing interests: not wanting to take the effort needed to care for a child who needs frequent medical care, or having an interest in the inheritance money of the elder parent. Not all family relationships are positive ones. According to Kuczewski, however, in reconsidering informed consent in a relational context, "the thinking and the values of the patient and the physician gradually take shape." Here the family takes part in the patient's narrative "of self-discovery that helps her to reconnect with her values and give them meaning as expressed in choices."[81] In a relational view of mutual respect, patient, family, physicians, nurses, and others share decision making—share the ethical exploration of what is the right thing to do. No one loses power.

Healthcare professionals and the agencies and institutions where they work have a great deal of power and authority invested in them: the knowledge and expertise of the professional, the ability and authority or a given technology, the procedures and rules of the agency, and the legal rules outlined by a society. These places of power often leave patients and families feeling powerless. Like Dax Cowart, the burned man who wanted to be allowed to die, and others who have written advance directives that are not enacted, they experience feelings of powerlessness. One of the participants tells of his cousin, a single woman of 65 years, who, after a heart attack, said she did not want to be resuscitated in the future. She then had a cardiac arrest and was resuscitated against her previously stated wish. Although she returned to her normal health and actually went on living her life in her own house for several years, she continuously spoke against being forced to accept unwanted emergency treatment. We hear her anger: "I'm absolutely livid about it—every day of my life!"[82] She had not been heard. No one had paid attention to her wishes. Because her decision had been hers alone, the fact that it was not given heed made her powerless. She could not depend on others to hear her point of view. She experienced anger and deep feelings of abandonment.

Professionals also feel the aloneness experienced by patients in independent decision making. In a research study, nurses, residents, and staff physicians were asked about overtreatment in the intensive care unit where they worked.[83] These professionals described these treatments, the regimes they were a part of, as torture, horrific, degrading, and so forth. There are many reasons given for the treatment, such as patient/family expectations, fear of litigation, the availability of a given technology compels its use, or it is easier to let someone else make the decision. But what is even more worrisome, Anne Simmonds comments, is,

> Gaining expertise in diagnosis, appropriate treatment, and use of technology becomes a way of avoiding or at least overcoming the feelings of powerlessness and failure in face of illness and death. Thus, for both doctors and nurses the antidote to feelings of powerlessness is "to do." It is easier to employ available technology in the face of im-

pending death, than to acknowledge our powerlessness over death. Physicians offer treatment aimed at keeping the patient alive. Nurses offer care aimed at keeping the patient comfortable. Both concentrate on the skill of doing procedures or interventions well. The desire to control death results in ever-increased intervention with ever-improved technology. Such a course becomes "automatic" and can lead to interventions that are inappropriate for an individual patient.[84]

Powerlessness is present when relationship is absent. When relationship is absent, doing something technical is, at times, the only possible response. The narrow focus on technical care, body systems, and laboratory tests, in the face of the human suffering of the whole patient, eventually dehumanizes both the patient and the caregivers; these people forget *who they are*. "Thus, for a physician," says Simmonds, "this approach supports an increasing separation of the patient's physiology from their humanity. With such an approach, the person with the power to make the decisions is the one furthest away from the patient, which allowed him or her to separate the patient as person from the care they are receiving."[85] Here, the power vested in the individual decision maker results in feelings of powerlessness. Separating physiology from personhood, separating persons from one another, may lead to inappropriate and dehumanizing use of power. Mutual respect in a relational sense holds the possibility of *re-powerment*, placing the power within the relationship where people meet people, and, in that meeting, *ethical action may be found*.

CONCLUSION

Lesley and François Paulette, on hearing that their son's pediatrician was planning to report their decision to the Department of Social Services, took their son, K'aila, and fled to a neighboring province. They knew the power of the social welfare agency, the power that would compel the police to come to their northern home and take their baby into provincial care. The parents were afraid they would lose their child,

so they drove through the night to stay with relatives to protect him. Would a relational approach to ethics—an attitude
of mutual respect—avoid the confrontational, fear-filled situation in which running away was the only way to dissipate
the power of the doctor, the welfare agency, and the police?

Would an attitude of questioning, an uncertainty about
appropriate action, have encouraged K'aila's parents and doctor to keep the conversation going? Perhaps others, an ethics
committee or a native healing circle, could have been invited
to join the exploration, not to ask *Who is right?* or *What is the
law?* but *What is happening? What are you going through?
What is the fitting response to what is happening?* Opening a
space of uncertainty to continue the conversation may have
allowed for reflection, a space that respects differences of opinion and belief and respects each other. It is respect for uncertainty that holds power in its place. This respect might have
allowed the sharing of decision making and sharing of power
without the horrific experiences of hiding and fear.

Mutual respect means, rightly, that each person has power
that is fundamental to human development. Mutual respect
means conversation, so that all sides can be heard. In such a
conversation, one's autonomy is fostered through gaining voice
and perspective, and through the experience of engagement
with others. What seemed to happen in *A Choice for K'aila*
was that both the parents and the doctor acted as independent and isolated decision makers—both taking the responsibility of commitment to obligations (parent to child, doctor to
patient) rather than taking responsibility for responsiveness
in relationships—for each other as well as for K'aila. The unit
of analysis was the individual rather than the relationship.
There was no space given to each to be powerful, to exercise
the power that rightly belonged to them. Mutual respect, with
its attention to interdependency, fostering the autonomy of
each other, both to self and other, and the holding of power in
a visible and humble way, might be a useful guide to reconsidering the choice for K'aila.

"Ethical behavior is *not* the display of one's moral rectitude in times of crisis," says nurse Myra Levine; "it is the
day-to-day expression of one's commitment to other persons
and the ways in which human beings relate to one another in

their daily interactions."[86] "The Chinese character for acupuncture means golden needles. For me," says physician Steven Aung, "this symbolizes that the needle is only a bridge between myself and my patients. It is a bridge built on compassion and the cultivation of physical, mental, and spiritual energy. This is what does the healing—not the needle. The really important thing is the relationship of trust and respect between healer and patient."[87] It is the business of caregivers to explore patients' reasons, and even argue with patients about the decisions they wish to make, because, says lawyer Robert Burt, people are connected to each other. Caregivers (doctors, nurses, and others) are human beings who are necessarily involved in a patient's or client's life, and so, "we have to negotiate together what our shared meanings are about, what it is that you want me to do or not to do. In fact," says Burt, "it is correct not only for me to say, 'Why do you want to do that?' but it is permissible for me to argue with you if I disagree, and to argue strenuously with you on a variety of grounds."[88] Myra Levine, Steven Aung, and Robert Burt point to mutual respect, a striving to make connections with others to express compassion by giving necessary care and treatment. Relational ethics means initiating and maintaining conversation, and it means that ethics is found in our day-to-day obligations and responses to one another.

In this chapter, we have discussed mutual respect from the perspective of interdependence, fostering autonomy, and the importance of attention to power. Mutual respect focuses on *how* we treat each other and ourselves, rather than the *why* of a particular treatment. As an action ethic, relational ethics looks to the way we *are* with each other as doctors, patients, nurses, families, or chaplains. We are participants by *being with*, rather than *being for*, as mere spectators who only observe, advise, or treat. Relational ethics builds on the premise that human experience is shared experience that leads us to understand ourselves as persons who are connected to others. Relational ethics attends to those connections that bind us together as humans. It is *how* we insert a needle, *how* we enter into conversation, *how* we show respect, or *how* we are with each other. Knowledge of ethical theories and principles is vital in this conception of ethics, yet such knowledge, alone, is not sufficient for ethical practice. In working from a relational ethic, we would not be content with watching a person die after making a fully competent choice to forgo further treatment; rather, it would be important for us *to be with* a person who is dying.

In reality, relational ethics is already practiced in the thoughtful way we treat students and colleagues, in the way we welcome babies and comfort elders, in the way we express compassion to both the suffering of patients and families, and in the suffering of caregivers who are faced regularly with human tragedies. This text gives language to the action that healthcare practitioners enact in their daily care for the persons who need their services and support.

NOTES

1. Knud E. Løgstrup, *The Ethical Demand*, trans. Theodor I. Jensen (Philadelphia: Fortress Press, 1971), 27.
2. Robin S. Dillon, ed., *Dignity, Character, and Self-Respect* (New York: Routledge, 1995).
3. *A Choice for K'aila: May Parents Refuse a Transplant for Their Child?* VHS, directed by Frances-Mary Morrison, with Peter Downie (Toronto, Ont.: Canadian Broadcasting Corporation, 1990). This video, used in research discussions, was developed from the point of view of the parents, and thus could be thought to be biased. The Interdisciplinary Research Group discussed the video at one of its first meetings and again at subsequent meetings. Concern was raised that the representation of the story in the video may have limited the group from understanding the actual situation in its completeness.
4. William Morris, ed., *The American Heritage Dictionary of the Ethics Language* (Boston: Houghton Mifflin, 1978), 1542.
5. John Macmurray, *Persons in Relation: The Form of the Personal*, vol. 2 (London U.K.: Faber & Faber, 1961).
6. Ibid., 118.
7. *Saskatchewan (Minister of Social Services) v. P. (F.)*, Dominion Law Reports (20 April 1990), 134-43.
8. See note 1 above.
9. Tom L. Beauchamp and James F. Childress, *Principles of Biomedical Ethics*, 4th ed. (New York: Oxford University Press,

1994).

10. Lesley Paulette, "A Choice for K'aila," *Humane Medicine* 9, no. 1 (1993): 13-7.

11. Ibid., 15.

12. See note 7 above, p. 134.

13. See Robert A. Burt, "Conversation with Silent Patients," in *Genetics and the Law II*, ed. Aubrey Milunsky and George J. Annas (New York: Plenum Press, 1980); Elizabeth Flager, Françoise Baylis, and Sanda Rodgers, "Bioethics for Clinicians: 12. Ethical Dilemmas that Arise in the Care of Pregnant Women: Rethinking the 'Maternal-Fetal Conflicts,' " *Canadian Medical Association Journal* 156, no. 12 (1997): 1729-32.

14. Proxy decision makers legally act in one of two standards: (1) the best-interest standard, which means acting in the best interest of the person who is not able to make the decision, or (2) the substituted-judgment standard, which means acting in a way the person would have if he or she had been able to make the decision.

15. See note 10 above, p. 17.

16. Ibid., 16.

17. Ibid., 16.

18. See note 5 above, p. 60.

19. Ibid., 61.

20. Sean Hand, ed., *The Levinas Reader* (Oxford, U.K.: Blackwell, 1989), v.

21. See note 10 above, p. 17.

22. Zygmunt Bauman, *Postmodern Ethics* (Oxford, U.K.: Blackwell, 1993).

23. Godfrey B. Tangwa, "The Traditional African Perception of a Person," *Hastings Center Report* 30, no. 5 (2000): 39-43.

24. See note 5 above, p. 66.

25. R. Melvin Keiser, *Roots of Relational Ethics: Responsibility in Origin and Maturity in H. Richard Niebuhr* (Atlanta, Ga.: Scholars Press, 1996), 78, 79. See also Mark J. Kuczewski, "Reconceiving the Family: The Process of Consent in Medical Decision-Making," *Hastings Center Report* 26, no. 2 (1996): 30-7, who suggests that the role of the family is to help patients discover their own values.

26. Christine Harrison, "Personhood, Dementia, and the Integrity of a Life," *Canadian Journal on Aging* 12, no. 4 (1993): 428-40.

27. See note 5 above. John Macmurray, *Reason and Emotion* (London, U.K.: Faber & Faber, 1962); Philip Conford, ed., *The Personal World: John Macmurray on Self and Society* (Edinburgh, Scotland: Floris Books, 1996).

28. H. Richard Niebuhr, *The Responsible Self: An Essay in Christian Moral Philosophy* (New York: Harper & Row, 1963).

29. Bruce Jennings, Daniel Callahan, and Arthur L. Caplan, "Ethical Challenges of Chronic Illness," *Hastings Center Report* 18, no. 1 (1988): S1-16.

30. Kenneth J. Gergen, *The Saturated Self: Dilemmas of Identity in Contemporary Life* (New York: Basic Books, 1991).

31. Seyla Benhabib, "The Generalized and the Concrete Other: The Kohlberg-Gilligan Controversy and Feminist Theory," in *Feminism as Critique: On the Politics of Gender*, ed. Seyla Benhabib and Drucilla Cornell (Minneapolis, Minn.: University of Minnesota Press, 1987).

32. See note 2 above, p. 295.

33. See note 2 above.

34. Robin S. Dillon, "Respect and Care: Toward Moral Integration," *Canadian Journal of Philosophy* 22, no. 1 (1992): 105-32, 122.

35. See note 1 above.

36. Anne Donchin, "Reworking Autonomy: Toward a Feminist Perspective," *Cambridge Quarterly of Healthcare Ethics* 4, no. 1 (1995): 44-55, 53.

37. Robert A. Burt, *Taking Care of Strangers: The Rule of Law in Doctor-Patient Relations* (New York: Free Press, 1979).

38. Robert Burt and Dax Cowart, "Confronting Death: Who Chooses, Who Controls? A Dialogue between Dax Cowart and Robert Burt," *Hastings Center Report* 28, no. 1 (1998): 14-24, 15.

39. Sally Gadow and Carole Schroeder, "An Advocacy Approach to Ethics and Community Health," in *Community as Partner: Theory and Practice in Nursing*, 2nd ed., ed. Elizabeth T. Anderson and Judith McFarlane (Philadelphia: Lippincott, 1996).

40. Carol Gilligan, "Remapping the Moral Domain: New Images of Self in Relationship," in *Mapping the Moral Domain: A Contribution of Women's Thinking to Psychological Theory and Education*, ed. C. Gilligan et al. (Cambridge, Mass.: Harvard University Press, 1988).

41. See note 22 above.

42. See note 38 above, p. 17.

43. Ibid., 19.

44. See note 34 above, p. 108.

45. See Vangie Bergum, "Ethics as Question," in *Extending the Boundaries of Care: Medical Ethics and Caring Practices,* ed. Tamara Kohn (New York: Berg, 1999), for earlier publication of ideas presented here; see note 34 above, p. 129, n. 3.

46. See note 34 above, p. 129, n. 3.

47. Ibid.

48. Keiser, *Roots of Relational Ethics,* see note 25 above, p. 70.

49. Karen Lebacqz, "Humility in Health Care," *Journal of Medicine and Philosophy* 17, no. 3 (1992): 291-307.

50. Hans-Georg Gadamer, *Truth and Method,* 2nd rev. ed., trans. Joel Weinsheimer and Donald G. Marshall (New York: Crossroad, 1989).

51. Hillman describes *daimon* as the "carrier of your destiny." James Hillman, *The Soul's Code: In Search of Character and Calling* (New York: Warner Brothers, 1996), 8.

52. Jon Amundson, Kenneth Stewart, and LaNae Valentine, "Temptations of Power and Certainty," *Journal of Marital and Family Therapy* 19, no. 2 (1993): 111-23, 114.

53. Ibid., 112.

54. Ibid., 121.

55. Oscar London, *Kill as Few Patients as Possible and Fifty-Six Other Essays on How to be the World's Best Doctor* (Berkeley, Calif.: Ten Speed Press, 1987), 38.

56. Carole Anne Taylor, "Positioning Subjects and Objects: Agency, Narration, Relationality," *Hypatia* 8, no. 1 (1993): 55-79, 69.

57. Philip C. Hébert and Michael A. Weingarten, "The Ethics of Forced Feeding in Anorexia," *Canadian Medical Association Journal* 144, no. 2 (1991): 141-4.

58. Joan Liaschenko, "Making a Bridge: The Moral Work with Patients We Do Not Like," *Journal of Palliative Care* 10, no. 3 (1994): 83-9, 88.

59. Oliver Sacks, *Awakenings* (New York: Harper Perennial, 1973/1990), 225, n. 104.

60. Annette Browne, "A Conceptual Clarification of Respect," *Journal of Advanced Nursing* 18, no. 2 (1993): 211-7, 213.

61. Carl E. James and Adrienne Shadd, ed. *Talking About Difference: Encounters in Culture, Language, and Identity*

(Toronto, Ont.: Between the Lines, 1994).

62. See note 58 above, p. 88.

63. See note 28 above, p. 58.

64. Bergum, "Ethics as Question," see note 45 above.

65. See note 4 above, p. 686.

66. Dianne Tapp, "Exploring Therapeutic Conversations Between Nurses and Families Experiencing Ischemic Heart Disease," (PhD dissertation, University of Calgary, Calgary, Alb., 1997).

67. Ibid., 201.

68. Ibid.

69. Keiser, *Roots of Relational Ethics*, see note 25 above, p. 82.

70. Ibid., 82 and forward.

71. Vangie Bergum, "Knowledge for Ethical Care," *Nursing Ethics: An International Journal for Health Care Professionals* 1, no. 2 (1994): 71-9.

72. See note 28 above.

73. Burt, "Conversation with Silent Patients," see note 13 above, 170-1.

74. Ibid., 171.

75. Leonard Angel, *Enlightenment East and West* (Albany, N.Y.: State University of New York Press, 1994), 44.

76. See note 34 above, p. 116.

77. Susan James, "With Woman: The Nature of the Midwifery Relation," (PhD dissertation, University of Alberta, Alb., 1997).

78. Humberto R. Maturana and Francisco J. Varela, *The Tree of Knowledge: The Biological Roots of Human Understanding*, rev. ed., trans. Robert Paolucci (Boston: Shambhala, 1992).

79. See note 40 above, p. 16.

80. Kuczewski, "Reconceiving the Family," see note 25 above, p. 30.

81. Ibid., 32, 34.

82. Interdisciplinary Research Group #3.

83. Anne L. Simmonds, "Reflections on Life and Death in a Technological Society: Experiences of Doctors and Nurses with Dying Patients in Intensive Care," (DMin Thesis, Toronto School of Theology and Emmanuel College of Victoria University, 1996).

84. Ibid., 109.

85. Ibid., 110.

86. Myra Levine, "Nursing Ethics and the Ethical Nurse," *American Journal of Nursing* 7 (1977): 845-849, 846.

87. Steven Aung, "Golden Needles of Compassion and Competence," *Feel Good Magazine* 3, no. 4 (1998): 8-9, 8.

88. See note 38 above, p. 15.

4

Relational Engagement

INTRODUCTION

In this chapter, we will explore a relational ethic from the perspective of a central theme of *engagement* among caregivers and with people in their care. Relational engagement is found in the shared moment in which people have found a way to look at something together. There is power in the experience of people who have very different experiences coming to understand something together. How do we engage with each other? How do we stand close to someone else—to understand someone else's experience and to recognize someone else's pain? In current healthcare, we are always concerned about the involvement of a professional with a patient. Often the concern is about over-involvement—standing too close. In this text, we are equally concerned about under-involvement and the disengagement that some say has led to a "humanitarian crisis," a crisis that harms patients and professionals alike.[1] The story of Dax Cowart, retold below, highlights the theme of engagement as a major theme of a relational ethic.

Ethical engagement between people in the healthcare environment requires intentional action. The word *engagement* comes from Old French, *engager*, meaning "to pledge or commit."[2] It is easy to see the correctness of this meaning of engagement when we think of one's personal life, such as to become engaged to be married. It is not as easy to understand commitment in the interaction between practitioners and patients or clients of healthcare, teaching, or law, where relationships are temporary and not chosen. Yet, responsible caregiving in healthcare situations includes engagement, and engagement includes suffering with another.[3] Healthcare workers' commitment to engagement is experienced in their practical actions of daily care.

Other meanings of engagement also give cause for reflection. Engagement means "to become enmeshed or interlocked,"[4] an ethical concern for both partners in the healthcare relationship. Being enmeshed has to do with being entrapped or entangled, which is often a worry in engagement. Entrapment or entanglement goes beyond the needs of the patient and the healthcare relation. Can there be a way to be engaged that is positive—a way to be together without being enmeshed? We have to have boundaries, yet it is not always clear where "my experience ends and yours begins." How does engagement between professionals and the people they serve become too personal, too intimate, and too involved? When is the relationship not personal enough? When is the healthcare relation engaged and ethical, and when is it non-engage (or over-engage) and unethical? What are the boundaries? What happens when one person does not like the other?

People are warned of the danger in standing too close, being over-involved, and overstepping professional boundaries. One professional nursing document directs attention both to over-involvement and to under-involvement, and to violations of boundaries.[5] It gives excellent examples for nurses to use in thinking about what appropriate involvement means. But even in outlining scenarios that demonstrate how the context and the particulars about each situation must be considered, the boundaries of appropriate involvement are still not made completely clear. Over-engagement (sexual, financial, or emotional boundary crossings or violations) or under-engagement (neglect and abuse) are clearly ethical issues, but other, less stark abuses (such as not listening to each other) are harder to define.

Schultz and Carnevale say that the ideology of modern medicine opposes connection in order to remain objective and prevent emotional hurt for either the professional or patient.[6]

How, then, should one be engaged in an ethical way? How can an engaged commitment be sustained in the reality of everyday healthcare practice in which resources, including available time, are limited, in which technology is a significant partner, and in which healthcare has become big business? The use of technology brings clearer attention to the possibility of over-involvement (ability to invade, go into, and alter people's lives) and under-involvement (mere technical performance) at the same time. Does the fact that strangers treat strangers lead to dis-engagement? How can the reality that the healthcare system is filled with strangers be experienced without feeling estranged or isolated? How can busy professionals have time for engagement with patients?

In this chapter, we develop the theme of *engagement* by exploring the activities that indicate how relational engagement is present. In the first place, we explore the possibility that a stranger can be a neighbor, one who responds as a neighbor would. The stranger, as neighbor, is seen as someone like oneself, a fellow human, with whom we can engage. We will use the Good Samaritan story to explore neighborliness as necessary for engagement. We propose that the reality of engagement includes both giving and receiving and, as such, allows for a sense of abundance where replenishment (receiving) occurs from involvement (giving) to others. Engagement allows us to newly perceive the realities of time and technology as factors in our lived world that can be filled or expanded, rather than only as outward commodities that can be lost. We will also explore *vulnerability*, an attribute often thought of only as a negative. Rather, vulnerability will be explored as a positive trait or a strength that is needed for ethical engagement to occur. The chapter ends with attention to the kind of conversation that encourages engagement in healthcare practice.

WHO IS STRANGER? WHO IS NEIGHBOR?

We have come to know that professional practice, in healthcare at least, is most often a relationship of strangers. No longer does the image of the rural family doctor, one who knows the patient in a companionable way as friend and neighbor, hold true. We often mourn the loss of this ideal of the healthcare relationship. Even if the image of the rural caregiver is a myth, we now talk of strangers treating strangers. Individuals, both caregivers and recipients of care, come from different communities, traditions, and cultures. Physicians treat hundreds of people they have never seen before—and will never see again. Nurses change from unit to unit, assigned to a number of beds or patients, not to specifically named people. Physiotherapists sometimes just treat the back or the neck, and pastoral care personnel are responsible for treating the soul. Lawyers and judges are also part of the healthcare environment— sometimes to clarify legal requirements or to protect from liability, and sometimes to make an ultimate decision regarding treatment. Yet, instead of accepting the notion of a stranger treating a stranger in a cold and distant way as a necessary characteristic of modern healthcare practice, we might reconsider how a stranger can be a neighbor. The story of Dax Cowart gives some clues on how to think about engagement between people.[7]

GATHERING AROUND DAX

Shortly after Donald Cowart came home from the Vietnam War, he and his father were involved in a tragic accident. The father died. Donald Cowart was left with severe, body-covering burns. From the very first contact with the people who found him, Donald Cowart asked to be allowed to die. Throughout his treatment, "Dax," as he wished to be called, described his pain as being so intense that it was like being in a torture chamber. He said,

> The tankings at the hospital were by far the most painful because a Clorox solution was placed in the water. Even though they gave me very heavy doses of morphine before the tankings, it was still as if alcohol was being poured over raw flesh. Then when I was raised out of the tank, the room was kept so cold that I felt as if I was freezing to death. They would then take me back to the room and even there the pain was so intense that I could do nothing but scream at the top of my lungs until I finally passed out

from exhaustion even knowing that this would do absolutely no good. This pain in the tank continued seven days a week, week after week after week.[8]

Dax wanted the treatments to stop. He wanted to be allowed to die.

The story of Dax stimulated many questions for our research group. We watched a video that showed Dax's tanking treatments, where the radio played loud music, where caregivers talked to each other, and where Dax's cries were seemingly not acknowledged. There seemed to be no engagement between Dax and his caregivers—he screamed and cried for them to take care, while they focussed on their work without talking to him. Several words and phrases, sprinkled throughout the transcripts of the IRG meetings, show the character and struggle of our discussions as we grappled with the issues Dax's story raised for us:

> *Poverty of values . . . manipulation . . . pillar of strength*
> *. . . power struggle . . . cooperative . . . allowed . . . hostage*
> *. . . some degree of normalcy.*

We heard Dax's caregivers and friends say, "We did everything we could imagine to help him," or "they did the best they could."[9]

The ethical questions we began to ask were: Is distancing of oneself, as helper, the only way to care for patients who are in extreme pain and who have bodies that are permanently disfigured (facial burns, loss of hands, blind)? Is it the person's suffering that stops one from listening and talking? When the focus of care was on a particular body part, as suggested in the words of a doctor, "I had trouble with the eye and hand," did Dax feel like he was treated like an object? Is death the ultimate evil? Does the talk of death raise fear for both patients and caregivers? Can caregivers be persons too? Can caregivers disagree with patients?

We felt that our questions went well beyond the facts of Dax's demand to die, his forced treatment, his suicide attempts, his rehabilitation, and his continuing iteration of injustice. It seemed to us, too, that our questions are more complex than patients' rights or professional duties. The questions asked began to focus on the relationship between Dax and his caregivers. Twenty-five years later, Dax says, "when I was in the hospital there were many reasons I wanted to refuse treatment, but one was overriding—the pain. The pain was so excruciating, it was far beyond any pain that I ever knew was possible, that I simply could not endure it. . . . That is why I wanted to die."[10] Now we hear his pain. Now we can talk to him about it. But, as healthcare professionals, we need to ask ourselves if lack of engagement led to the overwhelming sense of pain that Dax experienced? Could a "shared moment"—a moment of looking at that pain together—have helped to ease the pain?

THE GOOD SAMARITAN

The New Testament story of the Good Samaritan shows the importance of being a neighbor. The ideology of the Good Samaritan has become so universal that the term is given a place in the dictionary, defined as a compassionate person who *unselfishly* helps another or others.[11] The Good Samaritan story is about a man who was beaten, robbed, and left on the road to die. Both a priest and politician look the other way as they walk by this injured man. Then a man from another community, a Samaritan, comes along, stops, and, with compassion, gives first aid, transportation to a hotel, and pays the cost of the injured man's care.[12] Both the lawyer, who prompted the telling of the story, and Jesus, who told the story, agree that, of the three men, the Samaritan is the neighbor. He is a stranger but a neighbor.

The story is thought to be an example of an unselfish act (an act of selflessness), but another look at the story helps us to see the story in another light. The Samaritan picked up the injured man, took him to the hotel for care, and then continued on his way to attend to his own business. The Samaritan acted like a neighbor and helped another person in trouble, then carried on with the responsibilities and commitments of his own life. He became engaged with the injured man, gave of himself in time and money, *but did not give up himself in sharing himself.* One could say that the Samaritan, in his attention to his own humanity, understood himself as one like the injured man, and such self-understanding allowed the Samaritan to be full of compassion, attention, responsiveness, and self-fulfillment. The Samaritan was still a stranger, and, as such, was an independent person with interests and commitments elsewhere. Could thinking about the Samaritan as being "self-full," rather than being "self-less," be instructive? If one is self-full one is attentive to both self and other.

The healthcare encounter brings into focus a particular kind of relation that connects strangers together in meaningful and even intimate ways.[13] The practitioner comes with specific competencies and a commitment to exploring what needs to be done for *this* person (respecting autonomy, values, confidentiality, et cetera) who comes for care. In an engaged relationship, the patient or client also comes with willingness to discuss her or his healthcare in an environment in which trust is an essential ingredient. A concern about strangers treating strangers might, more correctly, have to do with treating a person as only a *problem needing to be solved,* rather than treating each other with compassion and respect as neighbors would. Charles Taylor discusses how the self-interested focus of modern life and the primacy of technological or instrumental reasoning (with its search for control and domination of life and death) leads to fragmentation of community life.[14] Fragmentation leads to a feeling of general malaise or indifference by many people to the needs of others. If a technical relationship is all that is needed, then it does not matter whether patients or professionals are identified as strangers. In a technical relationship, one doctor or nurse is interchangeable with another doctor or nurse (it is the white coat rather than the face of the person that counts), and patients can be identified according to disease (the heart patient in bed #1). On the one hand, when recipients of healthcare are treated as objects, as diseases, or as problems to be solved, then caregivers become objects as well—faceless practitioners who mechanically carry out their professional duties. When we distance ourselves from others, we lose out. That is when we burn out. As patients become objects, caregivers become objects too. Engagement, on the other hand, offers a way for practitioners to find meaning in their work and for patients to find meaning in their illness. Engagement offers a way to make meaning out of a tragic experience—a meaning that can only be found by each person in her or his own way.

Relationship *as engagement* is not contractual, as in a simple contract between equals in which each party negotiates from a position of self-interest. Nor is relationship paternalistic, with the professional making decisions for the patient. Nor is it independent choice in which the client or consumer, alone, makes the treatment decisions. Engagement between practitioner and patient is an encounter in which one party, the practitioner, is committed to respond as a neighbor to the person in need of care—to be a Good Samaritan. Through the experience of responsiveness to the needs of the other, the caregiver discovers and responds to the moral commitment of relationship.

Wilfried Lippitz describes the moral claim of the "other" as an obligation, "to discover *myself* as an *I* in my responsibility for the Other, to step out of the maelstrom of my own self-referential, economic existence."[15] The ethical self, the engaged self, the "You and I," is again recognized. The ethical relationship arises because one person elicits a response from another that springs as a moral impulse as Zygmunt Bauman notes.[16] "By addressing myself to another, I practice this responsibility, be it reluctantly or not. A total refusal of it would express itself through murder. Total acceptance of it would coincide with perfect love," says Adriam Peperzak.[17] While the priest and politician in the Good Samaritan story who passed by and ignored the injured man on the road did not murder the man, their lack of engagement could be thought an expression of lack of commitment to their own humanity, as well as the humanity of the injured man. Lippitz suggests that engaged action allows for the discovery of abilities not previously known: "The Other enables me to do more than I can do."[18] As Bauman comments, "Moral behavior is triggered off by the mere presence of the Other as a *face*: that is, an authority *without* force . . . it is precisely that weakness of the Other that lays bare my strength, my ability to act, as responsibility. Moral action is what follows that responsibility."[19] We do not need to see weakness, vulnerability, illness, and need as negative concepts; rather, they are natural rhythms of human experiences that need particular attention and care. Engaged relationships make it possible (not just necessary) to be moral.

To be engaged means that one responds to the needs of others. In this moral response, one does not lose oneself, instead, it could be said that one gains one's self—finds out what one is capable of. Engagement does not hold altruism (self-lessness) as the opposite of egoism (selfishness). Rather, engagement, as a characteristic of ethical relationships, requires attention to the self and the other at the same time. Could it be that selflessness is, in reality, disengaged relation? Engagement requires "self-fullness," a fullness of personhood, as "You and I"—an attention to the self and to the other at the same time. To act in an engaged way, both caregivers and recipients of care are *whole beings*, both self-interested and other-focussed, in what Dillon calls person-directed attention.[20] We propose that self-*full*ness instead of self-*less*ness is a necessary quality of the Good Samaritan, in order to be a neighbor rather than to be a stranger. Complete selflessness can lead to lack of relation, because there is a lack of wholeness.

WHOLE PERSONS

One of the participants in our research describes coming to know a patient, as a person, during her care of him during one evening shift. The nurse describes how, as the evening wore on, the man became more *three dimensional* to her, more of a whole person, rather than only a man with a high-grade tumor. She learned that this dying man was a collector of folk songs. Although he could barely speak, the patient said, "You have to come and see my folk song collection some time at my house." The card index, at the nurse's desk, contains all sorts of information, such as how many people it takes to get a patient out of bed, mouth care, diet, radiation treatments, size of tumor, et cetera. There is no place on the card to write about a patient's life event (his recent romance, his love of folk music). In a focus only on technology or technique, there is no place in the treatment plan for knowledge of unique personhood that supports building relationship. The uniqueness of the person is lost, and, in that loss, engagement too is lost.

In describing the situation, the nurse begins to question how caregivers can assist this man to make decisions about these very crucial last few months of his life if they only have information about his disease and treatments. In knowing more about the patient than just the disease, they can get a sense of what is important to him, what kind of information should be given, as well as when discussion of death is appropriate and when it is not. Perhaps, as Humberto Maturana and Francisco Verlela note, "everything we do is a structural dance in the choreography of coexistence,"[21] a kind of understanding of the difference between technical know-how and personal knowing. Knowing the patient as a person allows for sensitivity when sharing knowledge, a sensitivity that makes it possible for the facts to be presented to each person in an appropriate way. Caregivers modify their interactions constantly in how they share and how they give information. It depends on the patient. This sensitivity to others comes through being sensitive to ourselves.

Sensitivity to the patient, as a whole person, is shown in the experience of a young student caring for a man with sudden chest pain as recounted by a research group member. After calling for help and waiting for more knowledgeable professionals, the student stayed with the man and breathed with him to slow his breathing. By the time the experts came, the patient's chest pain was gone. Breathing with the patient, the patient and student together established a comfortable rhythm. Focussing on the person, a breathing person, rather than the problem, chest pain, may have helped. If we think of patients as a "heart," then they become a "heart" in the end. That is exactly what happens. When we become so fragmented in our approach (a person just being a heart), we tend to approach each other in a very impersonal way. When we become impersonal, we distance ourselves from other people as persons. Being *with* the person, as a person, is much different than meeting the person as a disease, as a heart, a chart, or a case study. The situation on paper is so flat—no dance, no rhythm, no music. If the card index does not have room for the qualities of the person, it is easy to fall into the danger of labeling.

Of course, labeling is helpful: this is the diagnosis, this is the problem, this is the dilemma. Yet labeling can also be isolating, indeed, objectifying, as "the appendix in room 5." Do we not also obliterate persons or create a distance between us when we use phrases like "these people." That is: "You have to give *these people* a chance." Labeling a group of patients as *these people*, as "epileptics," as "diabetics," or as "manipulative" depersonalizes them. The labeling of a person as being in a "persistent vegetative state" is, perhaps, an extreme case, in which the patient is no longer a person but an inanimate object, like a vegetable. Labeling objectifies the problem, as if the problem is the person. Labeling splits people apart, making it easier to choose "parts" of the person to know about. Labelling is an easy way to become impersonal. One cannot be expected to know everything about a person—there is always more to know—yet labeling often denies the fullness of the person. For example, a man in a forensic unit is more than a rapist. The task of caregivers is to see past the label and respect the dignity of all people in their wholeness. For people who are merely seen as labels, giving and receiving is more difficult, perhaps even impossible.

GIVING AND RECEIVING

How do we stay engaged? How can caregivers be present for each particular patient and still maintain their own sanity? We worry about our ability to "be there," for this patient, and for the next patient, and the patient after that, and then 10 years from now. There is a fear, and it is a substantial and important reality, that healthcare professionals do not have enough resources for engagement with patients, or even with each other. Resources are at a premium; there is not enough money for staff, for equipment, or for services. There is fear of personal and institutional depletion where resources (time, energy, and money) are limited and, in a special sense, nonrenewable. The fear of *depletion* is powerfully debilitating. When we speak of involvement or engagement of healthcare professionals with patients, families, or even with each other, the fear of running out of resources is great.

Professionals and patients who live with a quantitative notion of expenditure, even when they are referring to personal energy and emotion, perceive the possibility of eventually "reaching zero or even going into debt." This quantitative language is evocative, and reflects, in part, a competitive business ideology that is prevalent in healthcare today. If we were to use a different way to frame the resources of time and energy, we might come to consider the idea that, with more involvement (more giving and receiving), more replenishment is possible; the more reciprocity there is, the more one's reserves are resupplied. With such reframing, it might be possible to consider that it is in detachment, rather than in engagement, that depletion occurs.

Thus, burnout might be a companion of too much detachment and distance, rather than of healthy, effective engagement, in which both caregivers and the persons in their care receive, as well as give. Within such the paradigm of detachment, depletion occurs not only because resources are scarce, but also because one is unavailable to others (patients, their families, and other healthcare professionals), and, thus, unable to be replenished by *interaction* with them. Of course, there are situations in which giving and receiving in this way may be impossible—during emergencies, when particular physiological treatments are momentarily crucial, or when patients and families are reluctant to share with healthcare practitioners. And, of course, there are times when just too many things to do leaves one gasping for breath, physically and emotionally. We do not intend to minimize the serious and deleterious effect on patients and practitioners of the drastic environmental changes in healthcare funding. We intend, rather, to explore how engagement can occur in spite of the difficulties that are experienced.

The questions, then, to be addressed must be: How can we be involved in an enriching way? How can caregivers and those whom they serve be engaged in a way that replenishes both? Can engagement be nurturing for all participants in the healthcare relation? And, more importantly, what is our ethical responsibility to encourage engaged relations? These questions beg even deeper ones: What are the conditions necessary within the workplace of hospitals or healthcare agencies for reciprocity in relationships to be generated? Here we begin to see more clearly how problematic it is to separate the discussion of micro and macro resources as two different ethical concerns.[22] We need to consider how the institution or agency must be committed to fostering ethical relations in union with the caregivers. Ethical relationships are not only found at the bedside.

Let us examine an early experience of engaged interaction, one that easily images a nurturing mutually beneficial interaction—the mother-child experience of breast feeding. With breast feeding, the baby needs to take from the mother (through sucking) in order to receive milk, and the mother gives milk to the child (through nursing) in order to stimulate hormones that produce more milk. Only through the act of giving milk and emptying the breast can there be replenishment. At the same time, the mother also receives in her giving of milk. In response to the nursing by the baby, the hormones that are released in the mother's body not only stimulate the let-down reflex in the mother's breast, but also provide the mother with a sense of well-being and ease—a way to make endless child care demands more sustainable. Some might call this an *abundance* paradigm, where the more one gives, the more one is replenished, and the more one receives the more one is able to be involved and to grow. Such an exchange is impossible in a mode of detachment.

A story told by an administrator of a small long-term care facility tells of how reciprocal interaction made it possible for both caregiver and resident to be replenished.[23] The administrator made it a habit to "roll up his sleeves" and assist in feeding breakfast to the residents of the facility. Many of the residents had lost their ability to converse about their lives or even to recognize who was feeding them. The administrator, as caregiver, decided to find out more about the people to whom he was serving breakfast. Through research with the residents' family members and members of the community, he found out about the residents' previous lives—marriages, children, occupations, hobbies, and concerns. A story was written about each resident, which gave caregivers a way to communicate with residents about those things that had been of interest in their lives (that is, singing in the community choir, immigrating from the Ukraine, loving to garden). These stories created pictures of these residents as people who had character built into the lines of their faces that showed the treasures of their life's experience,[24] and brought their person-hood into sharp focus for their caregivers. Even without ver-bal responses from the patients, the administrator found that this personal knowledge encouraged person-to-person inter-action and made his time feeding the residents more reward-ing for him. It is easier now, he says, since he gets something back, perhaps only a vague smile or slight flutter of recogni-tion or even the taking of food, which reminds him of his own personhood and his shared humanity with the residents. This example demonstrates a move from objectification to engage-ment, a move that changes the whole experience.

These examples of giving food and nurturance remind us of the need to consider that giving and receiving are not only a private arrangement between two (mother and child; ad-ministrator and resident). Others give to the giver as well—the doting father or a family that visits. It is also true that the mother must have food and care in order for her to give at all, just as the administrator must have the time and resources for him to spend feeding the residents in his facility. Engagement requires support at all levels: micro, meso, and macro. The relational net expands. We are beginning to see where macro and micro decisions serve and require commitment to rela-tionship.

Lewis Hyde speaks of the work of the artist. He says the artist's work is a gift, "which moves the heart, or revives the soul, or delights the senses, or offers courage for living . . . [and] is received by us as a gift."[25] Healthcare workers, too, experience these kinds of gifts—not the commerce of daily life—but the gift that revives heart and soul, which occurs while attending a good birth or sharing in a good death. In giving and receiving, the gift continually shifts: receiving en-hances the capacity to give again. Here the linear version of giving is suspended: a circular nature of gifts becomes a real-ity. The healthcare relation as engagement offers the possibil-ity for being resupplied or replenished. The fear of loss of energy and other human resources loses its power.

If giving of the self is a commodity that can be lost, then one has to worry about it: *How much can I afford to give to this person today? Will I run out of the ability to care?* But if giving of self is a renewable resource that is replenished through giving, there is no loss. If, as we propose, engagement between individuals includes both giving and receiving, it is important to rethink the moral edict, "it is better to give than to receive."

WHO GIVES AND WHO RECEIVES?

It is a common belief of caregivers that it is better to give than to receive. Caregivers learn this truism early in their professional training. One of our research group noted, "As a junior pediatrician I was taught that you cannot allow yourself to get too emotionally involved because you will not be able to do your patient any good. The particular area of child abuse problems just blew me away. I was told to not let that happen . . . otherwise 'you ain't going to be any good'."[26] Healthcare professionals have generally come to believe in the need to develop a certain distance in relationships to patients, so that they are not seen as personally benefiting from the relationship. Or, more importantly, they worry that they may lose objectivity by becoming emotionally involved: by putting everything in strictly physiological terms, and making sure we have no personal physical reaction, we translate everything into "science." We are saved from embarrassment—supposedly. But the possibility for a personal relation ends, because the relationship is kept in objective terms. The belief that the professional is expected to be the giver is common; to not show their own pain or suffering so that they can be strong for the patient.

A pediatrician, a member of our research group, who cared for a child who had a defect that was incompatible with life, describes how uncomfortable he was in showing his emotion. The child lived about two months longer than was expected, and the family was in the nursery every day.

I was very much impressed by the devotion, the commitment, and the warmth of that family, and the extended family. . . . The day the child died, we wanted to keep the child alive until the parents came. I remember calling the parents and saying, "I think you should be here." The child

*died before the parents came in and I was in a cold sweat
as I had to approach these parents. I stopped them from
coming into the nursery to tell them that the child had
died. They accepted that and went in and held the baby.*[27]

The doctor felt that his discomfort had become apparent to
them, and that, in showing his emotion, his sadness at the
death of the child, he was letting the parents down. But, in
fact, the parents were not upset; they were ready and able to
support the physician—they wanted to support him. Many
caregivers hold to a notion of professionalism that suggests
that the show of emotion is inappropriate, as emotion may
cloud rational thinking and lead to unhelpful care. The worry
of being too close or too involved is serious. There may well
be a concern that closeness will result in patients becoming
too demanding—wanting more than can reasonably be given.
And there is rightful concern about damaging involvement,
as demonstrated in incidences of sexual abuse, or the inappropriate use of power or authority at the expense of the vulnerable.

The notion of reciprocity or mutuality is a difficult notion
for healthcare professionals, in that one prime impetus for
becoming a professional is the desire to do good for others.
The principle of beneficence—working in the other's (the
patient's) best interest—keeps the non-reciprocal nature of the
professional relationship alive. Yet it may be worthy to question whether or not the healthcare worker is the only giver,
and see if it is truly possible, in the end, to say who gives
what to whom. All that we give, as healthcare workers, comes
from the people to whom we give—so it becomes impossible,
finally, to say who gives what to whom. The moment one steps
out of mutuality, burnout and depletion become a danger. With
engagement there is less of a danger. We begin to see another
reason for burnout—giving without understanding and accepting what is given back. If we think that practitioners are the
ones who must give because we are the experts, the professionals, we do not (indeed, should not) receive from patients,
or even each other. Perhaps by openly acknowledging that we
receive as well as give, practitioners will be enabled to give

better care. Increased attention to mutuality and engagement with each other may lead to a new creativity in professional practice, decreased threat of lawsuits, decreased stress, increased self-confidence and pleasure, and, as Robbie Helmich Henson puts it, "positive growth outcomes resulting from shared . . . well planned choices."[28]

Often discussion about receiving from patients focuses on the inappropriateness of gifts. Yet professionals, in deep reflective honesty about what we get from relationships, recognize that it is not the gifts themselves, but in the spirit in which gifts are given, that the impact of reciprocity is experienced. The fact that the pediatrician shared an experience that occurred many years earlier gives credence to its impact and to the need to bring this notion of engagement into the discussion. The directed focus on either the recipient (as the individual in need) or the practitioner (as the source of knowledge and expertise) rather than the relationship *between* these people, may be part of the ethical dilemma. The patient often has important knowledge regarding his or her own care, and the practitioner may sometimes be in need of support from another. How are caregivers to be cared for?

Throughout the discussion of engagement, the issue of time was frequently raised. There just is not enough *time* in the healthcare environment for engagement. At one point, years ago, the fantasy was promoted that increased technology would give more time, but that notion has been quickly squashed. Technology does not save time or give more time. Time, or lack of time, is the major concern of modern healthcare.

TIME FOR ENGAGEMENT

Our research group considered the story of a man who went to a "time bank." He figured he had probably 50 years of life, which he exchanged for large bills. Then, to feel wealthier, he exchanged the large bills for smaller units, for seconds. He then had millions of seconds. Once he had this currency arranged in front of him, he began to worry and became obsessed with saving it. He drank his tea standing up in the morning, ran to the office, and got there much too early. By the end of the week, he had saved some moments. But, the end of the week still came, the next week started, and the saving of time didn't "carry over." The man realized this and began to regret his decision to hoard seconds. He longed to exchange the little seconds, the miserable things, back for years—but found that he couldn't. One day, he felt a draft, a breath of air past his face, and realized he could feel time passing, literally. He realized he objectified time and gave it too much reality. So he went to bed and never got up again.[29]

In real life, we also fear that time will "run out." In healthcare, there seem to be two things we worry about: becoming too involved, and not having time to become involved at all. A closer examination of the second may indicate that there is no danger of the first, because we're too busy. Time is so limited that we do not have enough time to sit and talk to patients. Of course talking and holding hands of themselves do not signify that we authentically engage with another, but the feeling that we are running out of time is so pervasive that practitioners do not have time for many things that they may want to do. But it is also a matter of what we do with our time. What we want to do may not take any more time, but it may require being in the situation in a different way. It may require having a different stance, offering a different kind of care. When we distance ourselves, everyone loses.

In healthcare it is easy to give in to the notion that we do not have enough time when patients are lined up in emergency rooms and when there are too many very ill patients in limited hospital wards. It is especially easy to think of running out of time when death occurs. We are so concerned about time passing—each day flies by, our birthdays come too fast, old age is upon us before we know it. And as time runs out, we lose. In ethics, when we focus on outcomes, as is the case with utilitarianism, we tend to lose touch with how we *act* in the process. For example, during pregnancy, if the focus is always the due date, then we tend to overlook what is actually happening—the changes that occur for the woman as well as for the baby.[30] In focusing only on the outcome, the birth, we lose the sense of the process and experience of pregnancy, of how complex being pregnant is, and how the relationship between the mother and the child is developing during that important time. When we focus on outcomes, whether it is on rights and duties, or on numbers of patients, we may forget ourselves as moral actors.

A member of our research group told a story of a meeting with a physician that took less than two minutes. In those two minutes, the physician was present to her and her situation. He introduced himself, apologized for keeping her waiting, and thanked her for coming to see him. He identified the problem (by use of ultrasound), which needed surgery, told her "the bad news," and told her that she could now, since the test was completed, empty her bladder, "the good news." He assisted her up from the examining table, waited for questions and concerns, and then showed her to the washroom. The physician and patient were engaged for two minutes, but two minutes was enough time. In contrast, another member told how a midwife's relationship with a woman took two or three meetings before there was a sense of engagement. We see that engagement is not time-limited. Perhaps there cannot even be the goal that "the patient will have a therapeutic relationship with the nurse," but, rather, that there needs to be a willingness to meet the person with an attitude of respect and attention.[31]

Although there is a great need for more time and resources to be made available to healthcare workers, this outward resource may not be the *only* answer. Time management or efforts to simplify activities may not be adequate to deal with our contemporary reality of busier and more hectic lives. Can engagement with each other in meaningful ways give us a way to respond to the frantic life of healthcare workers? Or will it only make things worse?

Perhaps the currency of engaged relationship found in the inner concept of the lived time of being *fully present* to the other person and to the *needs* of the moment is a useful way to explore the impact of time on relationships. Richard Niebuhr describes "time-full existence" as being present to the other in the encounter.[32] The time-full self is a "self that is always in the present to be sure, always in the moment, so that the very notion of the *present* is probably unthinkable apart from some explicit reference to a self, *I* and *now* belong together."[33] The time-full self holds within *presence, the being present,* the past, present, and future. Perhaps there is only one way to expand time: be fully engaged with each person in each moment.

If one is held in the grip of the past or the future, there can never be enough time, since one is already in two places at once. If, however, one is present with the other in an engaged way, Niebuhr notes, "past, present, and future are dimensions of the active self's time-fullness."[34] Here is the possibility that engagement expands time—at least for that moment. A relational ethic, as an action ethic, where persons are fully engaged in the moment, is "time-full in ways of which teleology and deontology seem unaware."[35] Anita Tarzian distinguishes between the Greek notion of nonlinear time (*kairos*) and chronological time (*kronos*).[36] With *kairos*, one remains fully present in the moment, to the point of losing track of time, or that time loses its demands. When we say that we "spend time" with patients, we may be focusing on a chronological sense of time. When we say that we "stay with" patients, we are focusing on nonlinear time, *kairos;* we have a sense of time stopping, or of a time that cannot be "spent." As Tarzian notes, "spending refers to attaching monetary value to an experience and exchanging units of equal value. *Waiting upon,* as a gift, cannot be spent or bought."[37] Practitioners, especially nurses, know that *being with* patients (in nonlinear time) at crucial moments will *save* (linear) time in the end. There is a rhythm in providing care—dealing with emergencies and their intensities and then dealing with the ongoing commitments to care.

Within a lived notion of time, depletion occurs when we are unavailable to be replenished by another. When we are detached, aloof, and distant we can give and not receive; detachment does not allow for reciprocity. Think of the intensive care unit (ICU), where patients are seriously ill and often dying. Anne Simmonds conducted research about the experiences of staff (nurses, residents, and staff physicians) regarding the over treatment (ongoing, continuous treatment) of dying patients.[38] The staff described their distress as feelings of

sadness, anger, depression, frustration, hurt, becoming dis-
heartened, or being empty inside. This moral distress, which
Simmonds found especially true for physicians, is thought to
relate to physicians who find themselves distant from the bedside, and whose distance does not allow them to experience
the possibility that death can be a positive experience. Often
in ICU medicine, death is experienced as the enemy, and the
technical approach tends to focus on body systems and laboratory tests, rather than on the whole patient. The bigger picture, the fact that the patient is dying, is sometimes lost in
this environment. The focus on the patients' physiology, on
organs or systems, separates patients from their own personhood and separates staff from their own humanity. Simmonds
says, "If the physician experiences the death of a patient as a
personal loss or narcissistic injury, then death becomes the
ultimate enemy to be resisted with all possible means; prolonging life becomes a form of self-protection."[39] If energy is
expended (*kronos* time) in self-protection, then there is little
left for engagement (*kairos* time) with dying patients—for listening to what patients say, through their bodies and through
their words about their wishes for their life and death. When
doctors and other healthcare practitioners are only attending
to the "parts" of patients, the possibility of burnout is great;
for when the part fails and death nears, there is no relation
between persons to enrich the experience of death.

We have learned from the ICU how the nature of the institution or unit shapes the care that is given and how it confines and regulates time. Where technology is pervasive, with
its monitors, intubations, and computers, it may tend to hinder
us from seeing the less obvious technologies, such as drugs,
intravenous lines, and blood pressure equipment, that distance people from one another. The techniques of assessment,
dressing changes, baths, and transfers, can completely hide
the need to attend to human meanings. Attention to technology can mask the reality of death, while attention to the reality of death reminds us of our humanity, in that death is a part
of life, and that there are limits to the skills, knowledge, and
actions of lifesaving treatments. The words human, humane,
and humility all come from the same Indo-European root,

dhghem,[40] which means earth, the ground of humanity. Being humane, being tied to the earth and its wonders, reminds us that humility is a valued characteristic. Karen Lebacqz says that humility includes reverence for, need for, and equality with each other.[41]

APPROPRIATE VULNERABILITY

One of the participants in our research notes, "There is an understanding in American Native tradition that the caregiver is required to both objectify the situation that he or she is in and also be part of it. Being part of it is the primary obligation and objectification allows the analysis."[42] In engaged interaction there is need for both objectivity (responsibility) and involvement (responsiveness). Standing back and observing is built on the scientific paradigm, while being a part of the situation comes from an ethical paradigm. The need to stand back and observe makes one humble—a state of mind that allows for continuous curiosity and a search for knowledge. Being present, as part of the situation, makes one vulnerable: We have to be prepared to embrace our own vulnerability in our relationships with patients.

Vulnerability is vividly experienced when a friend or family member is a patient. Dr. Ted Broadway relates that his friend has cancer and he finds that he has trouble letting her see his distress. "My patients have never seen my sadness and anxiety at their misfortunes," says the doctor. "Being a doctor seems to have indelibly altered my outward responses to this type of situation."[43] The doctor wants to remain calm and warm, and to never let his friend and patient see that part of him who wakens with wet face and heaving chest in the middle of the night. Yet the healthcare situation is often one of pain, suffering, and death, as well as healing, growth, and life. A fine balance is needed for caregivers to accept their own vulnerability in the face of daily human tragedy without being of no help to their patients or becoming overburdened themselves.

Acknowledging vulnerability (that is, bringing one's true humanity into the relationship) is closely related to the acknowledgment of emotion and the impact of power in relationship. If the healthcare professional experiences vulnerability, the experience of the power differential between professionals and patients is lost, and the possibility of engagement is expanded. Earlier we described what happened in the research group when one person shared a personal emotional insight in caring for a dying child. The emotion she shared made her vulnerable, and it made the rest of us vulnerable as well. We turned away. When we were *forced* by another research participant to discuss our discomfort, we began to uncover the belief that expressing emotion means being needful: *She needs help. . . . Something is wrong with her. . . . She has things to sort out.* We wondered, *What could or should we do? We are not her therapists.*[44] But do expressions of vulnerability need a professional to respond—to do something? Perhaps it may be that professionals—especially professionals, perhaps—need to rethink the belief that expressing vulnerability means neediness or weakness. Could we begin to see strength in such an expression of vulnerability? When we consider how vulnerability may be a strength, we may want to think about how caregivers can assist each other to face tough situations.

Engagement, as seen in the healthcare relation, is deliberate and is not based on likes or dislikes. Engagement is not an emotional response that overwhelms rationality and logic. As this is the case, engagement might be seen as differing from attachment. Attachment, defined as "to fasten, connect, or join" or even "to bind by personal ties or affection,"[45] may be more superficial and reactive than authentic engagement. One is attached or attracted to people whom one likes and detached or repelled from people one does not like. Engagement, on the other hand, requires reflection on how emotions, such as liking or not liking another person, are situated. Engagement encourages thoughtful deliberation about how likes and dislikes affect the possibility and responsibility of ethical engagement within relationships.

Ann Schweitzer's research talks about a situation in which she found that she intensely disliked a patient because of his history of wife abuse. She says, "As soon as I heard he abused his wife, I could not go near him. I came from a battered marriage—my first marriage—and I could not go near him. It was like you're the scum of the earth. As long as you're breathing, that is all that matters to me. I don't care if you are in pain."[46] The nurse was amazed at her reaction—a reaction she did not want to have. The reason she found her reaction astonishing was that her own experience of abuse had occurred 20 years earlier. Being curious about our responses (rather than judging them) invites reflection and gives us opportunity to engage with others in spite of our initial responses. To become engaged with a patient whom we dislike, we would need to be aware of *why* we have that reaction, and thoughtfully reflect on what we should do about it. Being honest with ourselves and the other person may be an important first step. Recognizing our own emotional reaction may release us from the emotional reaction of liking or disliking, so we can question how to become engaged with the person who is needing care.

Joan Liaschenko says that self-knowledge and reflection help to modulate responses to the patient: What kinds of issues do I have? What is this situation like for me? What is it about me that may get in the way of helping this person?[47] Understanding the self as a responsive being and interpreting responses such as anger, affection, disliking, or liking someone are fruitful in creating appropriate action. Engagement with another means that we are not ruled by passion or sentimentality nor by principles and rules, but rather by "a clear, distinct interpretation of all events as intelligible, rational events in a determined whole."[48] To wield emotional power, whether by liking or disliking, or by the cognitive power of expert knowledge over another person, denies human and rightful authority over our own lives, yet we are, to a large extent, inescapably dependent upon one another; in that dependency, we are also cognizant of the fact that we are in each other's power. As Lebacqz notes, appropriate vulnerability means having "a sense of our own limits and of our need for others [and] does not necessarily degenerate into self-abnegation, it can signal a healthy sense of community."[49] Engagement speaks to the community connection which needs attention.

Engagement between persons within the healthcare relationship, whether they are practitioners or people coming for care, requires conversation. The conversation or dialogue necessary for engagement moves past communication skill toward seriously addressing and responding to each other. Conversation, in this sense, is not easy. Yet conversation is essential for ethical relations in healthcare. Conversation makes relationship possible.

CONVERSATION

We began this chapter with the story of Dax, who requested that treatment be stopped and that he be allowed to die. Although Dax was considered able to be self-determining and to be cognitively capable, there seemed to be an attitude of nonengagement between him and his caregivers. Yet Dax, like every patient, has the right to be listened to, and if he had simply been listened to, he might have changed his mind. It might have ended up in hours and hours and days and days of talk, and that's what he had a right to have. He may, in the end, still have wanted to end his life. Until Dax was able to say "You are not listening!"[50] his lawyer friend was not able to admit his lack of attention. It is so hard to listen when someone says that they want to die, and wants someone to help them. There is so much at stake: the situation is full of fear for both. By listening, we ask the moral question *What is the right thing to do?* which can only be answered after hearing the responses to prior questions: *What are you going through?* and *What does your request mean?* Did Dax ask to be allowed to die because nobody would treat him as the man that he had become—because no one could face his pain, or confront his disfiguration, or listen to his screams, and realize what his experience meant to everyone involved? Do we, as caregivers, send patients on journeys to places where we would not willingly go? Do we, as caregivers, refuse to address our own vulnerability, especially when we are asked to accompany other persons to death? When the dying child or dying adult becomes a real person, it can be overwhelming for caregivers who see the pain and then stay in the pain. When we are totally aware of patients as "full" persons, we, ourselves are "full" persons—and that makes us very vulnerable. How can we do this?

Engagement is not possible without dialogue or conversation. But conversation is more than just verbal communication; touch, movement, the written word, and even silence have a place in dialogue. The focus of a relational ethic is not on defining a goal or ideal, and does not delineate a law or a duty; rather, it looks for the most fitting, most appropriate action for everyone involved in a particular situation. "Fittingness" is a concept that recognizes the complexity of interaction so that ethical decision making is not exclusively within the cognitive domain, but includes the way we speak, how we attend to the other, as well as how we interpret the situation. According to Melvin Keiser (who builds on Richard Niebuhr's notion of fittingness), a fitting response in moral decision making is one in which there is a "sensitive relating to the whole within which we are participating and to which we are creatively contributing."[51] Discovery of what is fitting or suitable requires compassion and responsiveness. The central paradigm for discovery of what is *fitting* is dialogue or conversation. Keiser describes conversation as responding in an appropriate manner to what is said to us—what we take the words to mean. While Keiser proposes that there may be many suitable responses, there are also limits to appropriate responses, but "we cannot lay out the limits beforehand; it can even be difficult to say afterwards what limit has been violated, yet we can sense it with confidence." Keiser says that while we do have ideas as we talk, they are more than just ideas: "It means more in the way we say things, the backing we give our words, the sounds and rhythms of our speech, the kinds of words we use as clear or ambiguous, simple or rich, and in the energy and intention with which we speak. Appropriate response in conversation engages these various aspects.[52] In conversation there is a give and take, agreeing with each other on some aspects and countering ideas with other ideas. Yet the give and take of ideas is only one aspect of conversation. There are other less tangible and less definable aspects expressed that show the fit of ethical decisions.

Dialogic conversation involves give and take, back and forth, being strong and being vulnerable, listening to stories of pain and staying in pain, and confronting death and staying with the dying. A relational engagement, through conversation, is not primarily interested in ideas, goals, or duties, but in persons in their particularities. It is not focused on reasoning, but is focused on trusting, feeling, and interpreting. Engagement does not occur with conformity to theoretically prescribed demands, but occurs creatively in the midst of concrete situations. It does not occur in linear or chronological time (*kronos*), that is, partial modes of time, future or present, but occurs in the fullness of time (*kairos*), which includes the past, present, and future. When conversation "breaks down," persons become things—a disease, a part, or a problem—and are obliterated. When patients become things, practitioners obliterated. Dialogic conversation, on the other hand, brings persons back into being—brings knowledge back to life.

Although some scholars in relational ethics bring a theological perspective, their insights are equally pertinent to a secular exploration of ethics.[53] Because relational ethics strives to discover what is fitting in each situation, there is little room for ideology or dogma. The language that is used in conversation gives a clue about the genuineness of engagement. As Keiser asks. "Is the language being used defensive or dialogical, commanding or collaborative, impositional or interactive, exclusive or inclusive, denying or affirming newness, attentive only to surface forms or as well as to deep mystery?"[54] Language that indicates that a conversation is taking place does not encourage conformity to an ideology (whether theology or scientific), but responds to actual people in their own life situations. To be a dialogical person requires us to aspire to authenticity (interpretation), openness (trust), integrity (accountability, and discipline), and responsiveness (intentionality).

Authenticity means being present with one's whole being, able to listen with heart and mind. The authentic person stays present—not attending to other tasks that lay ahead or are behind. Authentic persons recognize dependency (interdependency) as they are able to learn as well as teach, receive as well as give. Authentic persons recognize their independency (interdependency) as they know how to stand on their "own two feet," and have clarity around boundaries—about whom one is and whom one is not. In dialogue, authentic persons are able to engage with others without manipulating them.

The healthcare practitioner, as an authentic person, acts with steadiness and objectivity to converse with persons in her or his care, especially when the information that is shared is disturbing. The authentic practitioner chooses the facts and their implications most appropriate to the moment, which helps patients to deal with the realities of their own health or illness. Through dialogue, the meaning of the facts may change both participants. As Melvin Keiser notes, "We must wrestle with the immediate action to interpret what it means rather than sorting through our set of principles for the right one to apply. This struggle is always within a community of 'other knowers' so that understanding will involve articulate patterns communicated by and communicable to others. But the focus is on actuality rather than ideas."[55] The comprehensive knowledge required for the delivery of ethical care must include not only the facts, but their meaning for the people involved; further, these meanings may change and be enhanced by dialogue. This grasp of the meaning, the whole, is a creative process that is different than a law or a goal. Grasping meaning through interpretation must start from the particular situation, and progress to attending to it, working from it, toward new understanding. Authenticity cannot be achieved by having practitioners take acting courses to help them to convey "appropriate, beneficial responses to those emotional needs"[56] of patients, as some have suggested. To convey appropriate responses that "mask the physician's convictions, commitments, and attitudes may adversely affect the health interests of patients,"[57] and is the opposite of the kind of authenticity we are proposing. Engagement cannot be accomplished through courses in acting.

Conversation requires openness, in which one must be willing and able to reveal oneself to others and also be willing and able to accept others' revelations. Revelation, here, does not mean that one talks about oneself, but offers, in the conversation, a relationship in which meaning and vitality can be deepened. In a dialogic conversation, the hearer is as important as the speaker. *Listening is vital.* The hearer has, with listening, power to enable the speaker to say what needs to be said; in fact, to enable the speaker to discover what needs to be said, and, thus, to increase the possibility of understanding. Of course, the responsibility to listen and to hear is a mutual one. Reuel Howe comments, "Dialogic communication is the medicine for the loneliness that results from human alienation and separation."[58] Openness includes hearing the question behind the question, the fear behind the bravado, the insecurity behind the strength, and, perhaps most significantly, the courage behind the timidity. Healthcare practitioners, as experts in their own disciplines, bring, through engagement with the people they care for, responsibility and integrity that fulfils.

The healthcare practitioner in relational ethics is committed to assuming responsibility for self and others, and is willing to accept the limitations as well as the opportunities that engagement through conversation offers. There is a responsibility in conversation to prune the desire to talk too much. As we question the notion that available technology must be used, so too the dialogic communicator must watch the tendency to say something just because it is there to be said. At the same time, sometimes courage is needed to say what needs to be said, and to do what needs to be done. Failure to speak or to act appropriately is failure in responsibility. It takes courage to give ourselves to truth in its broadest sense and let that truth be acknowledged. One of the risks of conversation is the tendency of one person to carry both sides of the dialogue, assuming the correct answer and anticipating a certain response. Such cultivated monologue, which precludes speaking or responding freely, can be lessened if there is careful waiting for response.

Dialogic conversation fits easily within the notions of relational personhood and fostering autonomy. In relational personhood, the "You and I" are tied to one another, dependent on one another, as well as independent of one another. The particular is understood within the global—the person lives in an interdependent world. The dialogic word is an open word, a word of beginnings, because it is a word of expectation inviting response.[59] Relationships can fall apart, and dialogic conversations may be no more than an ideal, when relatedness is not accepted as necessary for flourshing human life.

CONCLUSION

How can one put such a notion of engagement into practice? How might we have stayed very close to Dax, in his story, to see him, hear him, or understand what was happening to him? If we stay that close, we are vulnerable to immersion in his pain and his suffering. So the question is, how do we stay completely present and not fall back on socially and culturally and psychologically acceptable coping methods, methods at our disposal for self-protection, things like distancing, leaving, reducing others' experience? We seem to be continually concerned about a lack of resources. There are not enough organs for transplantation, hospital beds, doctors and nurses, et cetera. The need for resources cannot be denied. Even in the example of breast feeding, if the mother does not have food, no matter how much the child sucks, the milk will run out. Even with the example from long-term care, if there are no interested individuals and resources available, the stories of people are lost, and the physiological characteristics of persons are the only ones given consideration. Even in the example of the ICU, if it is the expectation of both patients and their families, as well as staff, that it is necessary to do more and more to stave off death, then there will be no chance for engagement. Economic, political, and consumer issues are important. Yet, when engagement is an ethical commitment, we may change our understanding of what resources we are talking about, and consider how giving and receiving might moderate the demand to do more.

NOTES

1. Henry Abramovitch and Eliezer Schwartz, "Three Stages of Medical Dialogue," *Theoretical Medicine* 17, no. 2 (1996): 175-87; Ross Van Amburg, "A Copernican Revolution in Clinical Ethics: Engagement Versus Disengagement," *American Journal of Occupational Therapy* 51, no. 3 (1997): 186-90.
2. William Morris, ed., *The American Heritage Dictionary of*

the Ethics Language (Boston: Houghton Mifflin, 1978), 433.

3. Pellegrino says, "In the presence of a patient in the peculiar state of vulnerable humanity which is illness, the health professional makes a 'profession.' He 'declares aloud' that he has special knowledge and skills, that he can heal, or help, and that he will do so in the patient's interest, not his own." Edmund D. Pellegrino and David C. Thomasma, *A Philosophical Basis of Medical Practice: Toward a Philosophy and Ethic of the Healing Professions* (New York: Oxford University Press, 1981), 1; see also Dawson S. Schultz and Franco A. Carnevale, "Engagement and Suffering in Responsible Caregiving: On Overcoming Maleficence in Health Care," *Theoretical Medicine* 17, no. 3 (1996): 189-207.

4. See note 2 above, p. 433.

5. Alberta Association of Registered Nurses, *Professional Boundaries: A Discussion Paper on Expectations for Nurse-Client Relationships* (Edmonton, Alb.: Alberta Association of Registered Nurses, 1997).

6. Schultz and Carnevale, "Engagement and Suffering," see note 3 above, p. 190.

7. *Dax's Case: Who Should Decide?* VHS (New York: Unicorn Media for Concern for Dying, 1985).

8. Ibid.

9. Ibid.

10. Dax Cowart and Robert Burt, "Confronting Death: Who Chooses, Who Controls? A Dialogue Between Dax Cowart and Robert Burt," *Hastings Center Report* 28, no. 1 (1998): 14-24, 17.

11. See note 2 above, p. 567.

12. Luke 10:25-37.

13. Judith Ann Spiers, "The Dance of Caring," (unpublished master's thesis, University of Alberta, 1994).

14. Charles Taylor, *Philosophy and the Human Sciences,* vol. 2 of *Philosophical Papers* (New York: Cambridge University Press, 1985).

15. Wilfried Lippitz, "Ethics as Limits of Pedagogical Reflection," *Phenomenology + Pedagogy* 8 (1990): 49-60, 59.

16. Zygmunt Bauman, *Postmodern Ethics* (Oxford, U.K.: Blackwell, 1993).

17. Adriann Peperzak, "From Intentionality to Responsibility: On Lévinas's Philosophy of Language," in *The Question of the Other: Essays in Contemporary Continental Philosophy,* ed. Arleen B. Dallery and Charles E. Scott (Albany, N.Y.: State University of New York Press, 1989), p. 17.

18. See note 15 above, p. 55.

19. See note 16 above, p. 124.

20. Robin S. Dillon, "Respect and Care: Toward Moral Integration," *Canadian Journal of Philosophy* 22, no. 1 (1992): 105-32.

21. Humberto R. Maturana and Francisco J. Varela, *The Tree of Knowledge: The Biological Roots of Human Understanding*, 1st ed., trans. Robert Paolucci (Boston: New Science Library, 1987/1988), 248.

22. See chapter six for further discussion of the environment.

23. Joe MacGillivary, conversation with the authors, Edmonton, Alberta, 1996.

24. Catholic Health Association, *People of St. Mary's Health Centre, Health & Healing: A Review of the Catholic Health Association of Alberta & Affiliates* (Edmonton, Alb.: Catholic Health Association,1997).

25. Lewis Hyde, *The Gift: Imagination and the Erotic Life of Property* (New York: Random House, 1983), xii.

26. Interdisciplinary Research Group #4.

27. Interdisciplinary Research Group #2.

28. Robbie Helmich Henson, "Analysis of the Concept of Mutuality," *Image: Journal of Nursing Scholarship* 29, no. 1 (1997): 77-81, 79.

29. Interdisciplinary Research Group #4. The story was attributed to Rilke, but the specific source is unknown.

30. Vangie Bergum, *A Child on Her Mind: The Experience of Becoming a Mother* (Westport, Conn.: Bergin & Garvey, 1997).

31. Nellie A. Radomsky, "Creating New Meaning Through Dialogue: A Case Story of Chronic Pain and Sexual Abuse," in *Quality Culture: Quality in Turbulent Times*, ed. J. Ross et al. (Camrose, Alb.: J. Ross Enterprises, 1994).

32. H. Richard Niebuhr, *The Responsible Self: An Essay in Christian Moral Philosophy* (New York: Harper & Row, 1963).

33. Ibid., 93.

34. Ibid.

35. Ibid.

36. Anita Tarzian, "Breathing Lessons: An Exploration of Caregiver Experiences with Dying Patients Who Have Air Hunger," (PhD dissertation, University of Maryland, 1998), 180.

37. Ibid., 180.

38. Anne L. Simmonds, "Reflections on Life and Death in a

Technological Society: Experiences of Doctors and Nurses with Dying Patients in Intensive Care," (unpublished DMin thesis, Toronto School of Theology and Emmanuel College of Victoria University, 1996).

39. Ibid., 112.

40. See note 2 above, p. 1513.

41. Karen Lebacqz, "Humility in Health Care," *Journal of Medicine & Philosophy* 17, no. 3 (1992): 291-307, 299.

42. Interdisciplinary Research Group #3.

43. Ted Broadway, "Confusion Under the White Coat," (Toronto) *Globe and Mail*, 24 May 1994, A20.

44. Interdisciplinary Research Group #4.

45. See note 2 above, p. 84.

46. Ann Schweitzer, "Exploring Narratives of Relationship in Intensive Care Nursing," (PhD dissertation, University of Alberta, 1994), 80.

47. Joan Liaschenko, "Making a Bridge: The Moral Work with Patients We Do Not Like," *Journal of Palliative Care* 10, no. 3 (1994): 83-9.

48. See note 32 above, p. 58.

49. See note 41 above, p. 299.

50. See note 7 above. This statement by the lawyer was part of the *Dax* video.

51. R. Melvin Keiser, *Roots of Relational Ethics: Responsibility in Origin and Maturity in H. Richard Niebuhr* (Atlanta, Ga.: Scholars Press, 1996), p. 83.

52. Ibid., 82

53. For example, Reuel L. Howe, *The Miracle of Dialogue* (New York: Seabury Press, 1963); John Macmurray, *Persons in Relation,* vol. 2 of *The Form of the Personal* (London, U.K.: Faber & Faber, 1961), 157; Niebuhr, *The Responsible Self*, see note 32 above.

54. See note 51 above, p. 200-1.

55. Ibid., 89.

56. Hillel M. Finestone and David B. Conter, "Acting in Medical Practice," *Lancet* 344, no. 8925 (1994): 801-2, 801.

57. Ibid., 802.

58. Howe, "The Miracle of Dialogue," see note 53 above, p. 75.

59. Ibid., 83.

5

Bringing Knowledge Back to Life

INTRODUCTION

In this chapter, the theme of embodiment will have our attention. Embodiment expresses the recognition that people live in a specific historical and social context as thinking, feeling, full-bodied, and passionate human beings. Focusing on embodiment brings us back to life as we live it—that is, the integration of mind, body, and spirit. Embodied knowledge is not just the knowledge that we think about and discuss. Embodied knowledge is lived, in full subjectivity, through action. Of course, human existence is always an embodied existence—of flesh and bones and blood and pain, and in this chapter we will show that we enter relationship (action) in an embodied way. In fact, relationship cannot happen without embodiment. Relationship requires knowledge of both objective awareness (the thinking mind) and subjective awareness (the feeling body). Factual knowledge is not enough.

Embodied knowledge is revealed primarily through story—narrative—as embodied knowledge is found in life as we live it, feel it, and experience it. It is through narrative that we deepen our understanding of relational ethics. One of the special powers of stories is to recount the ineffable, the inexpressible, the things that can't easily be known. We propose that there is a need to value embodied knowledge as much as we value theoretical knowledge. Informational and analytical knowledge is particularly meaningful in the moment, and must be updated constantly. The knowledge found in story is different. This type of knowledge—sometimes called wisdom—is preserved, concentrated, and capable of being released as valuable knowledge months and years later.[1] Story avoids the coherent authoritarian voice used by scholars and experts, and reveals the variety of content, style, and views that are not usually made public through dominant theoretical traditions.[2] Such varieties may include views that Carole Anne Taylor describes as being "from the place I could not have thought [of]."[3] Story touches our hearts as well as our minds, and, as such, it is a most difficult thing. Sometimes it is extremely arduous to sit and listen to somebody's story—to the "unfolding of a lived life,"—as Robert Coles calls it, rather than listen to the facts that are necessary to prove a theory.[4] To develop relationship, we need more story and less theory. In relationship, we meet people in the flesh.

The wisdom of the story is particularly beneficial when we approach end-of-life issues, as death and dying create such fear within most of us that discussions of death are often avoided in the conversation of everyday life. Whereas dying was once a public process in the life of the individual, it has now, as Walter Benjamin described, "been pushed further and further out of the perceptual world of the living."[5] In the past, people were born at home, within the family environment, and died among the family, who often used the time of death to recount the story of the dying person's life. Now, in our modern lives, it is possible for people to avoid the sight of the dying, as death occurs primarily in institutions. Death is often thought to be the most disturbing and stressful of life experiences. Death, without the narrative unity of a person's story, seems to have become meaningless, the ultimate failure—a slap in the face for modern medicine—a failure of knowledge and a failure of technology. Our fear of death ultimately might be seen as a lack of relationship (with each other, with God, or with the universe). Yet, at the moment when death is near, the reality of relationship and the meaning of life presents itself in its depth. Death, be it our loved ones' or our own dying, is a time when the need for relationship and embodied experience with each other comes intensely to the fore. In this chapter, we begin our exploration of the theme of embodiment, the integration of body, mind, and spirit from its dualistic opposite, the split between body and mind and spirit—a split that has become a very deep chasm.

In this chapter, we will use the stories of two women who come close to death to illustrate the vital importance of embodied knowledge for ethical care: Margo, elderly and suffering from dementia; and Allison, young and brain-injured.

THE SPLIT

The dualistic body-mind split, frequently identified as the hallmark of the philosophy of René Descartes (1596-1650), is a subject of intense discussion and debate among philosophers, developmental psychologists, educators, and others. The split that we discuss here not only attends to the mind-body splits, but those splits or dichotomies that are reflected in other areas of life: the split between objective and subjective, between professional and personal, self and other, and between autonomy and community. Here we will discuss both the benefits and harms that are associated with these splits and oppositions, and propose that developing a relationship between the opposites can assist in creating new knowledge and understanding. To heal the splits and to move beyond the oppositions—such as mind and body, objective and subjective, or, indeed, self and other—we propose that we focus on the quality of the relational space that is found within these oppositions. The relational space begins with attention to intersubjectivity (where relationship is primary, and subjects are secondary)—where body and mind are distinguishable but inseparable, and where you and I are distinguishable, different, and individual but inseparable. The relational space, a space characterized by interdependence and interconnection, is, *at the same time*, a space where autonomy and independence can also exist. The assumption that autonomy and connection may occur at the same time is essential: we do not lose ourselves for the sake of the other; rather we find ourselves as fully autonomous persons through relationship with others. John Macmurray writes, "In acting I meet the Other, as support and resistance to my action, and in this meeting lies my existence."[6]

When knowledge is an outcome of participatory consciousness through relationship (that is, knowledge "in here" as different from knowledge apprehended "out there"), it (participatory knowledge) "requires one's full, somatic, and immediate presence."[7] When values (as experienced from within) and facts (apprehended from outside) are understood as inseparable, the questions *How do I know?* (epistemology) and *How should I live?* (ethics) can be understood as the same question. According to Macmurray, "If I do something, then I know that I do something . . . so thought presupposes knowledge, and knowledge presupposes action and exists only in action."[8] From this place of relationship (of action), we leave the flatland of dualism to develop knowledge that can give place to life in its deepest contours. Beginning and end-of-life experiences show the hills and valleys of life most vividly. Let us begin by gathering around Allison—a young woman at the end of her life. Allison's father and two sisters came to a meeting of our research group.[9]

GATHERING AROUND ALLISON

Allison Brown was a beautiful, young, active married woman when her car slipped off the road one rainy night as she drove home from work. After three or four months of intensive care, during which Allison did not show any signs of response or improvement in her consciousness (from the multiple, diffuse brain injuries), the neurosurgeon told Allison's family to put her in an institution, forget about her, and get on with their lives. Her family could not do that. Instead they had her transferred to an extended-care facility in her home community, which made it possible for her to have frequent weekend and vacation visits to her parent's home and with her family. Because there was no treatment available in the facility, the family recruited and trained volunteers to provide Allison with a consistent program of physical exercise and mental stimulation, which they thought useful for her improvement. Over the next four years, however, Allison did not improve. She never emerged from a persistent incognitive state.

The story of Allison and her family gives us opportunity to consider throughout this chapter the importance of lived reality of nonduality: the integration of body, mind, and spirit, and how this split, while valuable in some ways, is detrimental in other ways. The split between mind and body, with its celebration of reason, led to liberation from the dark ages of superstition, parochialism, and feudalism. It was through this split that art, mythology, morals, religion, science, and technology became fully differentiated. During this period of enlightenment it became possible to talk of self, culture, and nature as discrete and separate from each other. Prior to this development these domains were fused but not integrated. In fusion or immersion, questioning and reflection were not valued; indeed, they were not thought necessary.[10] Differentiation between the body (having a body of cells and functions), mind (having rational awareness), and spirit (living a life of meaning)—between having a body and being a body, between theory and practice, between subjective and objective, and between you and me—is a necessary step in our human evolution. Just as a baby must separate from its mother for both baby and mother to grow and become fully autonomous, so the development of our world is built on these differentiations, these splits.

Through differentiation and identification there have been spectacular advances in the empirical, technical, medical, and healthcare sciences that give increasing ability to order, arrange, and control nature and human life. This has been good. Scientific knowledge is essential. Yet we need to be careful not to *mis-place* scientific knowledge by letting it, as Raimond Gaita described it, "threaten our understanding of our creatureliness and of the way it enters our understandings of ourselves as human beings."[11] The problem comes when we begin to think that reduction and selection of ends is the only way to understand life, as if all aspects of life can be approached and described by these objective, narrow, scientific ends. The problem comes when we are forgetful of being— *being* in our bodies, *being* in our relationships, *being* in our world, and *being* in our universe.[12]

So our problem is not the various splits—the mind and body being the most famous. Rather, the problem arises when one is caught in the split. Coming from the Old Latin *capere*, "catch" is restraint or being trapped.[13] When one is caught in the split, one is unconsciously trapped in dissociation, separation, and isolation. On the one hand, if we identify only with the mind, we are left, as Ken Wilber said, with a map but no map-maker, a surface map of the world with no interior, the world of simple location.[14] In such a world, there are no interpretations, just facts; as Wilber says, "for surfaces can be seen, but depth must be interpreted."[15] In such a world relationships wane, meaningful living is forgotten, and individuals are "on their own." On the other hand, being identified only with body (matter) is also dangerous—the danger is that persons may be reduced to their biological function, of becoming just a heart or a number. Women, especially, have experienced the offensive and oppressive attitude of reducing the self as a whole to identification with one aspect of the self—the body. Many of us, both philosophers and healthcare professionals, have come to identify with the dominant world view of "I think, therefore I am" and to dualism, where the knower is, according to Macmurray "a pure subject, a mere observer, an isolated self, imprisoned in the fortress of his own ideas, and incapable of breaking out."[16] As we move from the attitude of "I think" to "I do"—to action—ideas are broadened and can change as they encounter the realities of everyday life.

DUALISM AND BIOETHICS

While the split between body and mind led to progress in many areas of life, it left us in peril as well. Through a discussion of a paper by a well-known philosopher, Helga Kuhse,[17] we will be able to see a danger that the theoretical split between body and mind poses to bioethics. In this paper, Kuhse is primarily concerned with the authority and usefulness of advance directives[18] in assisting with end-of-life decision making, especially with people who later suffer from severe and debilitating dementia. Discussion of the authority of personal directives to assist in making plans for dying exposes Kuhse's theory for understanding what it means to be a person.

Kuhse outlines a number of perspectives[19] as she focuses on a patient called Margo.[20] Kuhse reasons that people like Margo, who has severe dementia, are no longer persons. Her theory, which has considerable support from numerous philosophers,[21] argues that individuals/patients with dementia are no longer persons but are like animals: "They [animals] are not persons because they, like severely demented human individuals, lack the capacity for self-consciousness, rationality, and purposive agency, and have no concept of themselves over time."[22] Within such a theory, healthy infants (whose self-consciousness has not yet developed), people with severe dementia (who have lost their self-consciousness), and cognitively impaired children and adults (who never had and never will have such cognitive capacity) are not persons. As they have lost (or never had) a sense of personhood, patients such as those with dementia may be easily seen as objects (its) rather than subjects (he or she, mother or father, son or daughter). Sometimes it seems that there is less moral connection or commitment to objects than there is to subjects, although there are many who believe even things (objects) deserve our relational respect.[23]

In her paper, Kuhse emphasizes Margo's cognitive, rational ability rather than her ability to enter relationships. If we focus only on a property carried by an object (cognitive ability) rather than on an individual as a subject (able to connect to others or have others connect to her), there is no need to be concerned about embodiment. When we observe Margo as a cognitive object, we do not need to connect ourselves to her in a practical way: knowing her in a theoretical way is enough. With our theoretical knowledge, we hold Margo, as a cognitive object, at a distance from us. In this chapter, we will explore the possibility that a theory of personhood that is built solely on individualistic moral agency is a theory that can lead to insensitivity, and, if it is used as an engine of exclusion, can lead "to great wickedness," as David H. Smith called it.[24] A theory that leaves people alone in false states of isolation and alienation (states of harm) needs to be rejected. If individuals are treated as nonpersons, there is a danger that they may be treated as objects. And when one treats another person as an object, then real danger is seen: everyone may become an object. In treating others as objects, we all lose subjectivity and lose our moral capacity to affect and be affected by the other. When humans find themselves surrounded by nothing but objects, the result is loneliness, and, as Ken Wilber worried, this vast loneliness "has soaked into every strata of our society."[25]

Kuhse asks an important question: Who is Margo? This is also the question a young doctor, Andrew Firlik,[26] asks after visiting Margo during his gerontology rotation. Margo is cared for by an attendant in her own home. On his visits, Firlik says that he often finds Margo reading. She tells him she is particularly fond of mysteries, but Firlik notices that her place in the book jumps randomly from day to day. Although Margo does not seem to remember his name, she always seems pleased to see him. In her art class, Margo enjoys painting— the same circles in soft hues, day after day. She also listens to music. Indeed, she seems happy to listen to the same song again and again, as if she were hearing it for the first time. Kuhse and Firlik wonder: How does Margo maintain her sense of self? What happens to a person when he or she can no longer accumulate new memories as the old fade? What remains? Who is Margo?

Healthcare professionals, says Kuhse, "do not generally draw philosophical distinctions between persons and non-persons,"[27] and may find it emotionally difficult to withhold life-sustaining treatment from people like Margo. We agree with Kuhse that healthcare professionals cannot easily move away from direct contact with people in their care to develop an abstract philosophical theory. They cannot easily consider patients in their care as nonpersons, as if they were animals. For no matter how much we empathize with animals in distress, it will always be less poignant than our feelings for humans in distress. Raimond Gaita tells a story of driving behind a truck carrying animals to market, and how one would react angrily at the cruelty of seeing the animals held in small cages without water. But when one notices a child's face in one of the cages, it becomes a sight one would never forget.[28] Healthcare professionals are caught by the physical and social presence (the face) of the individual before them. Nurses talk about having to "be with someone." If the nurses are going to cope with caring for a person 24 hours a day, year after year after year, they have to be able to learn to see this person as a *person*.

For healthcare professionals, human beings with severe brain injury or dementia are still someone's mother, or sister, or, at least, someone's child—they are not an "it," an animal, or, as a member of our research put it, a "hunk of something."[29] Healthcare professionals are faced (from the work they do) with seeing the poverty of theories that base the notion of what it means to be a person on only one aspect of human life, such as the issue of cognition. Healthcare professionals touch and are touched by people like Margo, whom Firlik likens to a tree uprooted by a great storm. Margo, says Firlik, "compels you to cross the street, walk up behind her, and get ready to catch her in case an especially strong gust blew her off her feet."[30] The danger of a theory that defines some human individuals as "no longer persons" is that healthcare professionals and others *may no longer find it emotionally difficult* to withhold treatment from patients in their care. Rather, seeing the person in the fullness of human life (even with limited cognition) may make decision making at the end of life even more difficult (both rationally and emotionally) and, indeed, more burdensome.

Vikki Stark writes about her mother, Dorothy, who slowly lost her ability to be the lively correspondent she had been during and after her tenure as a vice-president of a New York public relations firm. After her move to Montreal, made so she could be closer to her daughter, Dorothy became more and more debilitated and not able to carry on her correspondence with her friends. It was then that her daughter began to write letters for Dorothy, "At first, I would read the letters to Mom while we were having lunch and get her to answer. I would scribble her responses on the back of the letter, then transcribe it at home and mail it." Later, Stark says, "I can't give up my job of writing back to her friends, my new pen-pals, and telling them what there is to tell about Mom. How she seems happy most of the time. How she exclaims with delight every time I turn up." In spite of the reality of Stark's own busy work and family life, she continues to visit her mother, reads her mother's letters to her, and responds to the letters. She enjoys "keeping the old Dorothy alive in writing back to those special women in New York."[31] The *person,* Dorothy, is kept "alive" through the letter-writing of her daughter and her friends. Although Stark writes about her activities as a pleasure, not a burden, it is not hard to picture the burden of ongoing commitment to letter writing as a challenge.

To heal the split between the mind and the body—that which occurs with the philosophical world view of "I think, therefore, I am"—is to develop a conscious awareness of it and to understand its potential danger. This consciousness is also found in the Latin root of "caught," *capere,* meaning to accept, anticipate, perceive.[32] The danger occurs when we, as human persons, no longer see ourselves as we really are—as both autonomous and reciprocal, as both rational thinkers and embodied beings tied to the world as we live in it. It is not a case of saying that either mind or body, either objective or subjective, is better or more accurate than the other. Rather, what is necessary is to recognize and hold the tension that is produced by flowing between these polarities. What is needed is to perceive what is at stake, consciously pay attention to it, and decide what is to be done. The tension between the two apparent truths should shift out into a larger truth that incorporates both. The challenge is to hold both in esteem, and, in that tension, find a greater truth.

Embodiment does not call for a return to unconscious immersion or symbiosis between mind and body, or self and other. Rather, embodiment calls for a healing of the split between mind and body that can leave us in a place of dissociation and isolation. By developing a consciousness awareness, we build our capacity to understand. And, through understanding that develops a reciprocal relationship between mind and body, between self and other, we are encouraged to breathe together, to act together, and to be in relationship. We hold the tension in a relational space. Embodiment is found and experienced in relationship.

MINDFUL BODY

It seems that one of the problems—an indictment of the state of our medicine today—is compartmentalization, in which we address a system, state, or an injury, but we don't address *a person*. We stay in the mind or in the theoretical. To heal the body-mind split, one is "compelled to abandon the theoretical attitude and to start not from the 'I think' but from the 'I do'; to adopt the standpoint not of the observer but of the participant; not of the thinker but of the agent," says John Macmurray.[33] When we start from "I do," from action, we are not dealing "with the isolated self, excluded from existence in the world, but with persons in dynamic relation, each an existing part of an existing world,"[34] as Macmurray notes. In the move from "I think" to "I do," we are involved in practice, in both thought and feeling, in doing and being, in a unity in which mental and physical activity are distinguishable but inseparable aspects. The result is embodiment. Embodiment makes it possible to establish communication as it acknowledges the "You" as the counterpart of the "I." Embodiment is in the concrete action of healthcare practice, in which mind and body/feeling intersect, and not in abstract theory, in which mind is given primacy. Embodiment enables us to find the strength to accept the reality that includes human suffering and death as a part of life. We see ethical commitment to the *and* between people—no matter what their cognitive ability may be.

Ethical commitments, such as a doctor's relationship with patients like Margo, can be demanding (even onerous), requiring, as James Olthuis writes, "sensitivity, flexibility, the utmost in care and vigilance—and certainly trust."[35] Developing a relation between the mind and the body, between you and me, recognizes the wholeness of the individual as a unique person, an autonomous person, while recognizing that each individual is a part of the whole of our humanity, our world, and, indeed, our universe. Integration asks us to move away from identification with the polarities of mind or body, self or other, and instead asks that we flow between body and mind as part of our way of knowing. This shift in focus—our choice as to where we put our attention—underlies our ethical responsibility. We can take responsibility for what we do by addressing the ambiguity and uncertainty that conflicting knowledge may present to us.

SHIFTING ATTENTION

John Macmurray's theory explains why both the thinking mind and the feeling body are important and relevant for addressing ethical issues.[36] Both embodied knowledge and theoretical knowledge are essential. Yet, theoretical knowledge, according to Macmurray, is derived from the actions of concrete, specific bodies in the world that *is*; theoretical knowledge is derived from embodied knowledge. Embodied knowledge, with feeling (touch) as its primary sense, gives direct awareness of the world, establishing concretely what is ourselves and what is not ourselves. In the experience of feeling—of physical touch—we are aware of resistance and the reality of a common shared space. Knowledge, in its embodied fullness, provides awareness of—attends to—both self and other in this relational space.[37] As we "feel" the other person in this common space, it is difficult to be immune to the effects our actions have on the other. Embodied knowledge sparks our attention in ways that theoretical knowledge, by itself, does not, and this attention, according to Michael and Abigail Lipson, shapes our intentions to act and guides our actions.[38] Our morality comes from how we attend to the world and to the other, and that attention decreases egoism and self-centeredness.

Attention changes awareness. One of the members of our research group told how after attending an ethics conference where family members had described their experiences of being with their dying loved ones, her ethical awareness opened up about "how we as professionals have distanced ourselves from our patients."[39] She described walking into her young patient's room on her first day back on the unit and noticing a picture of a horse on the wall near the child's bed.

On the picture was written, "Hope you are home for Christmas. From your sister." She realized then how she had distanced herself from this little girl (a severely abused child) in all kinds of ways. She realized how unaware she was of her ability to cope with the horrific truth that this girl was dying from sustained and deliberate abuse. The child became a person, not only a patient who needed careful and attentive care. The professional was no longer *only* concerned with the clinical needs of this child; rather she was brought face-to-face with the moral issues of how we treat one another.

By shifting our attention from self to other, there is room to learn more about the other person, as a person, which enhances the possibility of moral understanding. But this "temporary self-forgetfulness is not to be equated with loss of self," as Lous Heshusius puts it, or a state in which the capacity for autonomy is relinquished, but points to "the possibility of fundamental self/other unity in which egocentric thoughts, feelings, and needs are voluntarily released."[40] Such moral choice (attention) shapes our response and action (intention). For Macmurray, attentional awareness constitutes the awareness of the other and self in relation, which is an awareness of the difference between self and other. Within this awareness of difference through attention to the other, we cannot ignore knowledge of our own needs either, as we are one component of the relation to which "You and I" belong. Nor can we ignore our knowledge of the "space" we both inhabit and share.

Within the relational space, Macmurray says that the process of withdrawal and return is able to focus attention on the self and other in relation, by overcoming self-centered, egoistic motivations, and acting instead from an understanding of that relation. Through the process of withdrawal into reflection, we are able to return to action with the intention to act in relation to our newly accumulated knowledge of each other. Through engagement, as we gain more understanding of the other; we can reflect on own our actions to see if the intention that preceded them was appropriate. Did we have accurate knowledge of the whole situation and the other person? How do we respond ethically when our knowledge about patients and families is limited? We may know something about them, a little bit, enough to give technically competent care. But awareness that we do not have the whole picture allows us to come to know patients differently. The native healer sometimes has to move into the home of a sick person in order to treat. In coming to know the patient, we need also to come to know ourselves. Macmurray makes it explicit that increased self-understanding contributes to our ability to understand others, and his concept of withdrawal and return allows for change in the other, the environment, and the self. The capacity for transforming our ethical understanding lies, in part, in our ability to shift from our taken-for-granted view, to become conscious of our habitual point of view, in order to see from another perspective.

KNOWLEDGE FOR ETHICAL CARE

What constitutes valid knowledge for ethical action? Can intuition be counted as valid knowledge? How do we grapple with this question? There are different kinds or levels of knowledge (descriptive, abstract, inherent, or relational) that are necessary for ethical action.[41] In her work, Sally Gadow shows that these three kinds of knowledge, while distinct, build on each other through dialectic analysis, leading to knowledge that is comprehensive and complex.[42] Descriptive knowledge is subjective knowledge, based on exploring one's changing personal values, symptoms, and experience. Abstract scientific knowledge; medical, instrumental, and technical thinking; and rationality as reasoning build on descriptive knowledge of personal symptoms and values. Relational (or inherent) knowledge builds on both subjectivity (description) and objectivity (abstraction). It is developed through intersubjectivity—through conversation and dialogue between people.[43] Henry Abramovitch and Eliezer Schwartz characterize these levels of knowledge as three stages of medical dialogue: the personal meeting stage (subjective), the examination stage (objective), and integration through dialogue stage (inherent and intersubjective).[44]

With relational or inherent knowledge (integration through dialogue), rationality includes relational, moral values as well as values that have been identified by principles of theoretical reasoning. Walter Jeffko proposes that while *reason* is a fundamental universal human characteristic, any adequate theory of reason must apply to all essential human activities, and he suggests that instrumentality is only one mode of rationality.[45] Jeffko, following Macmurray, suggests that an inclusive understanding of human reasoning must encompass relational moral values, because all such forms of knowledge are needed to give ethical care. Neither descriptive knowledge (understanding personal, individual experience) nor abstract knowledge (clinical medical knowledge, as well as philosophical rationality) are comprehensive enough to ensure the delivery of ethical healthcare. Relational moral knowledge that includes subjective description and objective factual knowledge is needed. Many times it seems that we place our full attention on abstract or objective science and miss subjective knowledge entirely. From the point of view now proposed here, ethical responsiveness (or responsibility) is not ruled by either passion (subjective knowledge) or by reason (theoretical knowledge), but rather is, as Niebuhr suggests, guided by interpretation of "all events as intelligible, rational events in the determined whole."[46] Neither passion nor reason can be whole on their own.

Through integration of body and mind, in embodiment, the meaning of being *a person* is claimed through understanding the relational quality of self, other, and the context within which self and other are located. We know that we are born into a world of human connections—a physical, social, and moral world of connections.[47] As we grow and develop as individuals, we struggle to find ourselves, as autonomous selves, within this clear sense of human connection. As we grow and develop, we come to value both autonomy and community. To change our focus from individual autonomy to mutual relationship, we find that action becomes central, because action is necessarily relational. Action supports a shift from an emphasis on the thinking self (rationality) to the feeling body (corporeality). Action supports valuing autonomy and community at the same time. It is the essence of this concept of embodiment.

When we *think about* the patient Margo and her lack of cognitive ability, exemplified by her lack of capacity for self-consciousness, rationality, purposive agency, and seeing herself over time, we, like Kuhse, can propose she is no longer a person. Yet, when we *touch* Margo, as Firlik does, when we share her snacks, observe her painting, or remind her of common experiences, we are present to her and she is present to us in real life. This bodily experience, the resistance felt in bumping into someone, raises awareness of what is "I" and what is "not I," as Macmurray puts it, and makes the person present in a way that a thinking mind cannot capture.[48] This is an awareness of both the self, as a person, and the other, as a person, at the same time showing the common boundary shared by both. Embodied knowledge of both self and others lessens the possibility that we can ignore or be immune to the effects of the actions that are produced. Here we see the young doctor, Andrew Firlik, deeply attentive to the shared humanity—his response to Margo as a fellow human person. Through experiencing this relational space, Firlik can talk of what he learned from Margo, "the determination she had seeded in his mind" so that he looked forward to his visits with her, wished she could remember him, or even recognize him.[49] "I observed Margo, leaning into the winds of her disease, fighting them off; Alzheimer's blows a relentless course. So I cross the street. I become close to Margo. I wanted to catch her before the disease knocks her down."[50]

Philosophical theorizing that occurs outside the reality of daily life benefits from the opportunity to gather around Margo and around Allison Brown. Let us listen again to Allison's family.

The first ethical decision the family made was to remain part of Allison's life, to support and love her. In fact, her sister says, they became engrossed in her life. Another ethical decision, which emerged out of the situation at that time, was to simply treat Allison as another member of the family, as an equal, different now than she was before her accident, but still a member of the family. The family always spoke to her as if she understood, and they believed that there was some meaning to her movements. They said that their ethics did not evolve out of abstract principles, or out of Allison's moral agency, but evolved out of the practicalities of what they were facing everyday. The final ethical decision was made four years later, after much discussion with family, professional staff, caregivers, and ethicists. At this time the family decided to remove the feeding tube that was keeping Allison alive.

For Allison's family, the dignity of human personhood (both of Allison and each member of her family) is rooted in the reality of relationship, rather than *only* in the properties possessed by one of the parties, whether that is cognition or moral agency. When death was near, the problem of relationships and the meaning of life were acutely experienced. The personal relationships between patient and doctor, family and healthcare professional, and family and the healthcare system were highly important. Through these relationships, the professionals and the family accompanied the patient to the end of her life.

EMBODIMENT SPACE

Embodiment calls for relational space. This relational space, space between body and mind, between self and other, is referred to as a *third space* by Homi Bhabha,[51] or a *dialogical space*, by Carole Anne Taylor,[52] that builds on the embodied reality of life as lived. It is in relational space, this relational reality, where opposites cease. This relational space is highly *contoured*, one in which we are on top of the mountain (rationality) and in the valley (corporeality) at the same time. From this reciprocal space, a solid place in the world where we live, we can draw from all aspects of life: our rationality, our emotionality, our connection to each other, our differences, and our grounding in the world. From here we can explore and develop the *quality of our relationships*, not only the quality of our minds or the quality of our bodies. From a relational view, morality and ethics begin with "responsibility rather than [individual] freedom, corporeality rather than in arguments, in pain rather than in concepts," as James Olthuis writes.[53] A relational view does not negate autonomy or a commitment to individual moral agency, but places both directly in the context of human relationship.

Attention to the feeling body, the body that is affected by suffering and by death, is a hard place to *be*, especially for healthcare providers who encounter life's tragic moments so frequently. Healthcare professionals have learned, or have been distinctly taught, to be objective and to keep emotions controlled in order for rational objective thinking to have full sway in decision making. One participant in the research group said,

> *If the truth were told, I immediately go into an objective mode because I'm extremely uncomfortable with that kind of emotion [that is, tears]. It's not that I don't feel it, and I can recognize this when counselling across the table. When someone comes and gives me a rational discussion, I know that if I kick him on the ankle, he's going to burst into tears. So I can feel these things, but I just feel uncomfortable. I even feel uncomfortable with silence.*[54]

The relational dialogical space, where feelings and emotions are valued, is not an easy place to be.

Relational space can be burdensome when we find ourselves in the midst of difficult and challenging ethical demands, and we are faced with difference: difference of values, beliefs, opinions, life experiences, cognition, functions, and abilities. In fact, it is difference (with its inequalities) that is central to our current moral reality. We must honor and respond to difference without breaking community. As Olthuis says, "Indeed, genuine community begins with the acknowledgment of difference."[55] Relational space asks us to consider what mutuality means, what mutual respect means. Taylor asks us to create a dialogical space where we position each other as subjects—subjects to each other.[56] We must change, Taylor says, from positioning others out of our own ideologies, our own dominance, our own hubris, where the privileged subject always appropriates others. Relational space calls for engagement with one another, for without engagement the patient is alone, no matter how many professionals are present.[57] Relational space requires embodiment, as a member of the research group said, a space to

> ... *understand and accept my own pain and vulnerability as mine and the others' pain and vulnerability as their own. That's crucial. It is crucial to know whose is whose so that I have to deal with mine in order to be able to stay present. And my emotions and reactions to another can*

signal to me the edges between us that aren't clear. It is
where I may need to pay some attention lest I be tempted
to reduce the person to an object.[58]

In a dialogical, relational space, we are asked to let go of the
assertive, explanatory address that values clarity, consistency,
and coherence, to include, as Taylor says, more "interrupted,
disjointed, or overlapping narratives to reflect changes in sub-
ject-position."[59] Further, Taylor notes, engaging in dialogue to
include all voices "renegotiates narrative and social power,
including what conventionally stands as coherence, judgment,
evidence or value."[60] With the changing multicultural landscape, there is a need to acknowledge the reality of whose
position, culture, gender, religion, race, and so on, is central—
and whose is marginal.[61] Taylor says that the multicolored
fabric of a world makes it necessary to "take a great deal of
collaborative effort for those in positions of dominance to work
through sundry forms of appropriation and complicity toward
social change."[62] To view difference as more than opposition
alters power relations themselves, and allows relationship to
be of primary importance. Relationship to others (as embodied whole persons) is the root of the matter—based in the practical, complex, discordant, incredible world in which we live.

James Orbinski, a Canadian and past president of Médicins
Sans Frontières (Doctors without Borders), delivered the 2001
University of Alberta Visiting Lectureship in Human Rights.
Dr. Orbinski told horrific stories of war. In one, he talked of
the 1994 murder of hundreds of Tutsi children in a Rwanda
orphanage. He talked of seeing butchered children whose bodies, soaked in blood, were left in a field. Prior to this genocide, Dr. Orbinski had attempted to negotiate for the release
of the children to a safe place. He was not successful. In the
course of the conversation with one of the murderers, he asked
the man if he had children. This man replied that, yes, he was
the father of four. But these, said the man, are not children,
these are insects and will be crushed like insects. Two hundred children were murdered, and "now lay covered by a blue
plastic tarp, in a heap of limbs and clothes, and blood that
made a brown-red mud of the soil beneath them. My most
stark memory of Rwanda is not of mass graves or the political

theory underlying the International Convention in the Prevention and Punishment of Genocide, but of small sausage-
like fingers—severed fingers—lying in the mud beside that
blue plastic tarp."[63] When asked how he managed to keep going after being witness to a situation like that, he said, "I keep
going by continuing to do what I need to do—by action in
order to keep the humanitarian space alive."[64] Keeping the
relational space open between us as people, as whole persons, allows us to keep our humanity alive. Viewing another
human being as a commodity, an animal, or an insect opens
the door to violence, hostility, and loss of feeling or indifference. We need to think about how we are all complicit in the
events like these.

Let us again gather around Allison Brown. What do we do
when our fellow human is reaching the end of life, through
loss of cognition, through loss of cellular function? Zygmunt
Bauman suggests that *all* we have is the "moral party of two"—
the quality of our relationships.[65]

Allison's family said that their ethics emerged out of a
family consciousness, out of the context of their situation, the
practicalities of what they were facing every day. They said
that their decision to withdraw the feeding tube was made
because they felt that Allison was caught in a kind of death,
yet, at the same time, she could not die. They came to know
that she did not want to be in her body: "We felt this intu-
itively." Her body was living, it served as an anchor to life,
but she wasn't really "in" it: "There was nothing behind her
eyes." They said that, as a family, they had to cut back on
their extensive involvement in the daily care that Allison
needed. They knew that in the hospital there would be very
little interaction and meaningful activity in Allison's life (only
time to turn, feed, bathe—asking staff to get Allison into a
chair was just too much). Without the family's care, Allison's
only alternative would just be to lie and wait. They said,

> This was a very big issue for our family. We felt that re-
> moving Allison's feeding tube was a spiritual act. Every
> member struggled with their conscience and then we came
> together many times to express our thoughts and feelings
> on how we could reconcile our intentions and Allison's
> wishes [expressed prior to her accident], and with our own

spirituality. We felt that it was the most difficult decision that we would ever have to make in our lives and we asked for spiritual guidance, not only from ministers and priests, but most importantly from within ourselves. Interestingly enough, members of our family had developed very different belief systems over the years—so we're talking Christians, Buddhists, New Ager's, and an atheist thrown into the mix, so we came from divergent beliefs. Yet, when it came to Allison, our beliefs converged to a general agreement about the meaning of Allison's life to her and the act of her death. Our convergence was actually gentle and after talking and talking and talking about it, we finally all agreed. We felt that our decision was correct based on who we were and what we knew of Allison.

The day we asked to have the tube removed, we told her what was being done. We treated Allison as if she were still a daughter, a sister, a wife, and a woman. We told her about our doubts and said that we were asking for spiritual help to make the right decision. Even though we were in anguish, she gave no evidence of her own. We had doubts, and there were times when we wanted to run into that room and say to put that tube back in but we still felt that this was the right thing to do. We were told that all great ethical decisions involved doubt and that this was something we were just going to have to live with. It came as part of making this decision. Our circle was then enlarged to include nurses, doctors, ethicists, ministers, priests, extended family, caregivers, and volunteers. It was this small community that gave us support and encouragement. They knew what Allison's life was like for the last four years, and they were there for her when she passed away.

The family and community decision about removing the feeding tube occurred in the mid-1990s. Some people might question why it took the family so long to make this decision. Some might feel that the family should have acted on Allison's wishes earlier. The family struggled to understand her wishes and to act on that understanding of her wishes. Allison's sister recalls the time they discussed Karen Ann Quinlan's story, which they had read about before Allison's accident. "Allison had asked me if I would please pull her tube in similar circumstances. I said, 'Sure, if that ever happens. Yeah, I'll do it. No problem.' Then I had asked her if she'd do the same for me and she said, 'I don't think so.' And I got really angry and said, 'Well, what do you mean. If I'm going to do it for you, why can't you do it for me?' And she said, 'I can't promise that I would be able to do that for you.' " For Allison's sister and her family, this discussion is one that gave them permission to do it or not to do it—when the time came. In fact, the family said, that it is "a curious kind of synchrony" that they had actually had this discussion.

It took four years for the family to come to the decision to remove the feeding tube. They said, "If anyone had recommended to us in the first two years to let her go, we would have thought, 'Oh my God, no! There's just no way we can do that.' But during the last year, we began to wonder whether enough good could be done for her in the future to justify what was actually being done to her now. We came to the unavoidable perception that we were increasing her suffering in order to keep alive the slim hope that she might get better, or to keep alive the hope that she was leading a meaningful and dignified life." The decision to remove the tube was a spiritual decision. At one point a physician had suggested that the family take Allison home and remove the tube themselves—not telling anyone. But the family could not do it. They believed that she should be surrounded by all the people who loved her, and not just family. They felt that deceptions and lies would have resulted in Allison dying without the love and affection of her friends, family, and the nursing staff. When Allison's family was deeply reassured and became committed to letting her go, they felt the right way to do it was for her to be surrounded by people who loved her. They felt that Allison would be able to "feel" the difference if her leave-taking was surrounded by lies and deception. She would take in or understand the atmosphere in a different way. It is a spiritual concern—that Allison could know things even when she was in a persistent incognitive state.

Action, in commitment to the dignity of each person through our relationships, is the only way to heal the split of our modern world, the split between mind and body, the isolation between self and other. It is the saving power. A community of knowledge is only possible through the community of action, the moral impulse that is called forth by touch and fed by thinking. Ethical action is the relationship between us, held by the deep respect for human dignity and difference. *Who is Margo? Who is Allison? Who is the family? Who am I?* Knowledge cannot exist in a void; it must be *somebody's* knowledge.

CONCLUSION

The relational space is the place where we dwell, a space that has been exemplified by Allison, her family, the professional staff, and volunteers who cared for her. The relational space is a dwelling place that nourishes both thinking and feeling, both objectivity and subjectivity, and both self and other. Here we can be together in difference and diversity; here we can find irreducible respect for each other as whole person—a place that is diversely colored, multistranded, cohesive, and strong. It is a place where we know each other. We do not go into a situation knowing and giving this perfect care. To be aware of that and then to move to a better level of care is to be ethical. The reflection and the self-awareness are part of being ethical because the most ethical practice cannot happen by just being technically competent.

We know that there are many people who are not in relation—who do not have a committed family like Allison Brown or a concerned doctor or nurse as Margo did. We know this from our own practice where patients are alone day after day—with no family visiting. We know this from the ongoing stories of sexual abuse of children. We know this from the gunning down of teenagers in our schools. We know it from hearing of horrific atrocities of war. But that is our task, is it not, as persons, as healthcare professionals, to recover the sense of relation between us—to stay involved and spend time with each other, with our patients—time that is respectful and extensive? It is enormously burdensome for a caretaker to take on a relational commitment, but this is the heart of caretaking, the heart of nursing and medicine, as Dax and Robert

Burt note.[66] It is the heart of healthcare. The tree of knowledge
is a tree whose trunk integrates and supports both the branches
and the roots. Without the trunk, the tree will die. Relationship integrates the knowledge of both thinking and feeling—
knowledge of body, mind, and spirit. Without relationship,
humanity will die.

NOTES

1. Walter Benjamin, *Illuminations* (New York: Schochen
Books, 1969).
2. Carole Anne Taylor, "Positioning Subjects and Objects:
Agency, Narration, Relationality," *Hypatia* 8, no. 1 (1993): 55-80.
3. Ibid., 70.
4. Robert Coles, *The Call of Stories: Teaching and the Moral
Imagination* (Boston: Houghton Mifflin, 1989), 22.
5. See note 1 above, p. 94.
6. John Macmurray, *Persons in Relation*, vol. 2 of *The Form
of the Personal* (London U.K.: Faber & Faber, 1961): 209.
7. Lous Heshusius, "Freeing Ourselves from Objectivity: Man-
aging Subjectivity or Turning Toward a Participatory Mode of
Consciousness?" *Educational Researcher* 23 (1994): 15-22: 20.
8. See note 6 above, p. 209.
9. Interdisciplinary Research Group #10. The story of Allison
Brown (not her real name) was shared by the family who gave
permission for the story to be used in publication.
10. Sally Gadow, "Relational Narrative: The Postmodern Turn
in Nursing Ethics," *Scholarly Inquiry for Nursing Practice: An
International Journal* 13, no. 1 (1999): 57-70.
11. Raimond Gaita, *Good and Evil: An Absolute Conception*
(London,U.K.: Macmillan Press, 1991), 127.
12. Brian Swimme, *The Hidden Heart of the Cosmos: Humanity and the New Story* (Maryknoll, N.Y.: Orbis, 1996).
13. William Morris, ed., *The American Heritage Dictionary
of the Ethics Language* (Boston: Houghton Mifflin, 1978), 1520.
14. Ken Wilber, *A Brief History of Everything* (Boston:
Shambhala, 1996).
15. Ibid., 245.
16. See note 6 above, p. 208.
17. Helga Kuhse, "Some Reflections on the Problem of Advance Directives, Personhood, and Personal Identity," *Kennedy*

Institute of Ethics Journal 9, no. 4 (1999): 347-64.

18. An advance (personal) directive is a document that may be comprised of: (1) a set of written descriptions of the type of healthcare an individual does or does not want to receive at the end of life; and/or (2) the identification of an agent who is the individual(s) whom one wants to make decisions on his/her behalf. In Alberta, when signed and witnessed, these documents carry legal authority and come into effect when an individual no longer has the capacity to fully participate in the decision-making process.

19. Kuhse discusses: (1) the precedent autonomy view of Ronald Dworkin, who argues that a patient's critical interests take precedence over merely experiential interests; (2) the psychological view of personal identity of Derek Parfit, questioning whether Margo is the same person she was before her illness as she is during her illness; and (3) the nonpersonhood approach of Allen Buchanan, which Kuhse favors. Allen Buchanan, "Advance Directives and the Personal Identity Problem," *Philosophy and Public Affairs* 17, (1988): 277-302; Ronald Dworkin, *Life's Dominion: An Argument about Abortion and Euthanasia* (London, U.K.: Hammersmith, 1993); Derek Parfit, *Reasons and Persons* (Oxford, U.K.: Oxford University Press, 1984).

20. Andrew D. Firlik, "Margo's Logo," *Journal of the American Medical Association* 265, no. 2 (1991): 201.

21. The philosophers Kuhse refers to include Dan Brock, Allen Buchanan, Derek Parfit, and Peter Singer. Dan Brock, "Justice and the Severely Demented Elderly," *Journal of Medicine and Philosophy* 13 (1988): 73-99; Allen Buchanan, "Advance Directives," see note 19 above; Allen Buchanan and Dan Brock, *Deciding for Others: The Ethics of Surrogate Decision Making* (New York: Cambridge University Press, 1989); Derek Parfit, "Reasons and Persons," see note 19 above; Peter Singer, *Practical Ethics* (Cambridge, U.K.: Cambridge University Press, 1993).

22. See note 17 above, p. 359.

23. Brian Swimme and Thomas Berry, *The Universe Story: From the Primordial Flaring Forth to the Ecozoic Era—A Celebration of the Unfolding of the Cosmos* (San Francisco, Calif.: Harper, 1992).

24. David H. Smith, "Seeing and Knowing Dementia," in *Dementia and Aging: Ethics, Values, and Policy Choices*, ed. Robert H. Binstock, Stephen G. Post, and Peter J. Whitehouse

(Baltimore, Md.: Johns Hopkins University Press, 1992), 47. It is not hard to remember great world tragedies resulting from treating marginalized groups—such as women, Jewish people, Blacks—as non-persons.

25. See note 14 above, p. 33.

26. See note 20 above.

27. See note 17 above, p. 362.

28. Animals are not, of course, exempt from moral consideration, but we know that our relationships with animals are different than they are with human persons. Gaita, see note 11 above, p. 117.

29. Interdisciplinary Research Group #7.

30. See note 20 above, p. 201.

31. Vikki Stark, "Writing Dorothy Back to Life," (Toronto) *Globe and Mail*, 30 March 1998, A24.

32. See note 13 above.

33. See note 6 above, p. 209.

34. Ibid.

35. James H. Olthuis, ed., *Towards an Ethic of Community: Negotiations of Difference in a Pluralist Society* (Waterloo, Ont.: Wilfrid Laurier University Press, 2000), 3.

36. See note 6 above. Macmurray's theory of the self is explored in Vangie Bergum and MaryAnn Bendfeld, "Shifts of Attention: The Experience of Pregnancy in Dualist and Non-dualistic Cultures," in *Globalizing Feminist Bioethics: Crosscultural Perspectives*, ed. R. Tong, G. Anderson, and A. Santos (New York: Westview Press, 2001).

37. John Macmurray, *Self as Agent,* vol. 1 of *The Form of the Personal* (New York: Harper & Brothers, 1957).

38. Michael Lipson and Abigail Lipson, "Psychotherapy and the Ethics of Attention," *Hastings Center Report* 26, no. 1 (1996): 17-22.

39. Interdisciplinary Research Group #4.

40. See note 7 above, p. 18.

41. Vangie Bergum, "Knowledge for Ethical Care," *Nursing Ethics, An International Journal for Health Care Professionals* 1, no. 2 (1994): 71-9.

42. Sally Gadow, "The Dialectic of Clinical Judgment," in *Clinical Judgment: A Critical Appraisal*, ed. H. Tristram Englehardt, Stuart F. Spicker, and Bernard Towers (Dordrecht, the Netherlands: D. Reidel, 1979).

43. See note 2 above.

44. Henry Abramovitch and Eliezer Schwartz, "Three Stages of Medical Dialogue," *Theoretical Medicine* 17, no. 2 (1996): 175-87.

45. Walter G. Jeffko, *Contemporary Ethical Issues: A Personalistic Perspective* (Amherst, N.Y.: Humanity Books, 1999).

46. H. Richard Niebuhr, *The Responsible Self: An Essay in Christian Moral Philosophy* (New York: Harper & Row, 1963), 58.

47. Raymond Duff, " 'Close-up' versus 'Distant' Ethics: Deciding the Care of Infants with Poor Prognosis," *Seminars in Perinatology* 11, no. 3 (1987): 244-53.

48. See note 37 above.

49. See note 20 above, p. 201.

50. Ibid.

51. Homi K. Bhabha, *The Location of Culture* (London, U.K.: Routledge, 1994).

52. See note 2 above.

53. James Olthuis, *Knowing Other-wise: Philosophy at the Threshold of Spirituality* (New York: Fordham University Press, 1997), 132.

54. Interdisciplinary Research Group #5.

55. See note 35 above, p. 134.

56. See note 2 above.

57. See note 10 above.

58. Interdisciplinary Research Group #4.

59. See note 2 above, p. 64

60. Ibid., 74.

61. See note 35 above.

62. See note 2 above, p. 73.

63. James Orbinski, "University of Alberta Visiting Lectureship in Human Rights," Edmonton, Alb., 6 March 2001 *http:// www.ualberta.ca/~lecture/2000transcript.htm.*

64. James Orbinski, conversation with Vangie Bergum, Edmonton, Alb., 7 March 2001.

65. Zygmunt Bauman, *Postmodern Ethics* (Oxford: Blackwell, 1993).

66. Dax Cowart and Robert Burt, "Confronting Death: Who Chooses, Who Controls? A Dialogue Between Dax Cowart and Robert Burt," *Hastings Center Report* 28, no. 1 (1998): 14-24.

6

Creating Environment

INTRODUCTION

Relational ethics is not something that can be reduced to a principle, but is the creation of an environment where ethical reflection can take place. In this chapter we propose that environment, as the space for ethical action, is not only something "out there" to be manipulated, but also the moment-to-moment, everyday occurrences that we live. In this sense, environment is created by our everyday action. It is an ethic for the present, yet it is an ethic that creates and protects the future. Through our exploration here and our reading together, we are working toward a kind of ethics that is situated in daily life. What we present, in an attention to relational ethics, is already among us in many instances, and very far from us in others. But even when it is operative, attention to relationship is often hidden within the dominant view of ethical discourse. As before in this book, we will bring the relational view through story; in this chapter we will discuss the decision that Joanna and Paul must make about whether or not to carry Joanna's pregnancy to term. In this discussion we will need to include various aspects of our dilemmas: the age-old as well as the modern factors (as discussed in chapter two) that are ever-present in any ethical decision. Relational ethics does not reduce complexity; rather it makes the complexity more apparent and then embraces it.

The ethical immensities of our world, especially our health world, often focus on issues of cloning, the status of the embryo or fetus, reproductive technology, resource allocation, transplantation, end-of-life issues, disability, research issues, and so on. Yet the ethical immensities of our world are also found in moments where we experience ethical complexities individually—in each decision we make about transplantation, each termination of a pregnancy, each decision to insert or remove a feeding tube, each time we consent to a particular treatment, or each time we neglect the suffering and oppression of others. Sometimes we have time to think about each momentary ethical decision. Sometimes, though, these ethical moments of decision making catch us unawares and compel us to ethical action before we have time to think or reflect—before we can even catch our breath. In such moments, we breathe in ethical tension and breathe out ethical action. We act because the immediacy of the moment demands it of us. We act from our embodied and theoretical knowledge of normative ethical theories, community expectations, virtues that we hold, knowledge of the law, understanding of our world, as well as our personal experience. In the immediacy of the moment we replace objectivity with dialogue, and we replace principles with relationship. These ethical moments create environment that integrates the micro and the macro— where the community ethos of equality and solidarity is held as surely as the focus on the individual situation. It is clear, given the dehumanization of the world (for the sake of the marketplace), the exploitation of the body (for the sake of perfection or preventing death), the depersonalization of medical care (for the sake of autonomy or professionalism and its ever-increasing technology), the alienation from each other (for the sake of personal wealth and individual freedom), and the revenge on those who are violent (for the sake of a sense of security or even for the sake of righteousness), that a new paradigm is necessary.

But a new paradigm, a relational paradigm, can only be put into action by considering how environment is affected by the immediacy of each ethical moment. Understanding environment in this way would be asking healthcare professionals to consider the personal as well as the abstract or scientific when they enter a room with a patient. We wonder how the system would change if we had healthcare professionals who were always able to do that. Oftentimes, when we discuss a relational ethic with healthcare professionals, the questions that surface are: a lack of time, a lack of resources and staff, and the debilitating effects of using the financial bottomline as an outcome measure. These facts are the reality of the healthcare environment. Could this environment change if attention to relationship was our primary ethical commitment? At the same time as we open space for a relational ethics, we are not limited to attention only to the individual relationship, but must include attention to the increasing social and divisive inequalities in the larger world. As Solomon Benatar writes, "In order to foster social cohesion that is required to advance the health of all people at national and global levels," we need to reconsider again the relationship between the micro and the macro.[1] We still have freedom to choose the direction we wish to develop.

FREEDOM AND CHOICE

Often, we hear that the pace of the development of technology has outstripped our ethical questioning about it, as well as our ethical understanding of the issues at stake. This seems true at both the individual level and the societal level. We also have come to accept that, in a democracy, our commitment to individual human rights gives us the freedom to make individual choices about how to live. Choice is necessary in our individual, social, and communal life. Individual choice is a value to cherish. Yet we need to think about how to put our moral beliefs into that field of choices, so we can make decisions in which common welfare, justice, and equity are given equal weight with individual rights and personal virtues.

In one session of our research, we explored the use of prenatal testing in helping parents to make a decision about the health of their potential child. While technology has opened up an infinite field of choices, we began to wonder how technology shapes the type of decisions that are made. As moral choices are not based on scientific or technical knowledge, but are based on commitment to the moral equality of all humans to live in an environment (be it a healthcare system or the world) where all can flourish, we need to explore how choices are made. Because the language of technology and science tends to obscure the lived reality and suffering of human life, there is a need to recover a more multivalent language that is richer in its symbols and poetic quality, to see what is needed for ethical action. While technology does not deal with human meaning, the ethical choices that technology opens enable individuals and societies to consider important and broad issues of human meaning.

GATHERING AROUND JOANNA AND PAUL

In 1992, the National Film Board of Canada produced a series of videos, "Discussions in Bioethics." One episode in the series, called *Who Should Decide?* describes a young couple, Joanna and Paul, who undergo routine prenatal diagnosis.[2] As the story unfolds, it becomes clear that the unborn child has spina bifida, and the parents have to decide, almost immediately, whether the pregnancy will be terminated. In the video, the doctor gives no direct guidance in assisting the parents to decide what they should do. She does, however, book a date for surgery "just in case." Joanna, an active, healthy working woman, wonders what the next step should be. She herself uses a wheelchair, as she, too, has spina bifida. At one point, Paul is seen talking on the phone with his parents; he avoids telling them about the unborn baby's diagnosis. Paul has already felt his parent's disappointment regarding his marriage to Joanna because of her disability. Joanna states clearly that she wants to have this baby, who, they find out through the ultrasound, is a girl. Paul is not so sure. In a poignant moment, Paul tells Joanna that he just wants to have a normal child—not a genius, not a professional athlete—just a normal child. Joanna asks her husband to tell her, *just what is normal? Who is normal?* For her, she says, not being able to walk is normal. For her, the life she has is normal. Joanna recognizes that it will be difficult for her to give birth and care for this child without Paul's support. She does not want to have this child alone. At the end of the video, Joanna says to Paul, "It is up to you."

Who should decide? Should it be the mother? Should it be the father? What part, if any, should the husband's parents play in this decision? What about the need for support from the grandparents in the care of a child? Should the doctor just give the facts (as she knows them) and then leave the parents to make the decision for themselves? By scheduling a surgery for termination of the pregnancy, does she already suggest a course of action, or is she just being expedient? It seemed that the doctor did not open space for the possibility that the parents might wish to have this baby. Should the parents have made a decision before having the test? Is it possible, rationally, to make a decision prior to the experience of having this test? What should the limitations of testing be—if any? What about the attitudes and expectations of the community for parents to have only "normal" children? What is a "normal" child? There are so many questions to consider as we gather around Paul and Joanna and consider the complexity of their decision. It seems clear in this situation that they, the parents, are the ones to make the final decision, yet other people will affect, and will be affected by, the decision that they make. To consider only the parent's relationship and their individual decision in this situation is not enough. First, though, let us explore informed choice, which is so important in ethical decision making. In the following discussion of informed choice, we suggest that comprehended choice may lead to more effective, as well as a more demanding, understanding of decision making. Informed choice and informed consent build on relational commitments, personal ethics, professional ethics, and legal obligations. The decision that Paul and Joanna will need to make considers all of these.

INFORMED CHOICE

The basic ethical commitment of respect for others requires that we do not do things to another person without their consent. Indeed, health professionals have a duty to give individuals reliable and adequate information so that they can make informed choices. As far as is possible, any decision involving consent should be a participatory one, based on the other's comprehension of the issue. True informed consent requires the patient to be actively involved. As such, we contend that the concept of informed consent falls short of the better concept of comprehended consent, and even further short of the best concept, namely, comprehended choice. Only informed consent, and its focus on individual choice, has recognition in law. Health professionals know that information is always incomplete, and that comprehension of what is known is also incomplete. In fact, health and medical care are practices in uncertainty, in spite of all the things that are known. Yet there is the ethical obligation to strive for a shared understanding with people before subjecting them, with their comprehended consent, to any treatment that carries any kind of risk of any sort (physical, emotional, or social). The risks as well as the benefits of a particular treatment or therapy need to be shared with those who are needing such care.

For consent to be valid, individuals must be mentally competent, be given information that is adequate for them to choose between treatment options (including doing nothing), and to know about the attendant risks and probable outcomes. Choice must be "free"—that is, it is free from incomplete disclosure; it must be framed in language that the chooser can understand; the chooser must not be subjected to undue persuasion or manipulation or influenced by possible conflicts of interest on the part of careproviders. For patients to make comprehended choices, they need to be involved in reasoned discussion of all of the options and open to consultation for second or third opinions with other professionals in complex situations.

Another important concept in informed consent concerns the domains of competency. Competency is not "all-or-nothing." Individuals may not be competent in one area (for example, handling their personal finances) and yet be quite capable of making decisions about their health. Competency, therefore, may need to be assessed for each domain of daily living. Further, competency may fluctuate, as ability to make valid decisions may waver in any day or time period. Decisions should be postponed until the decision makers have the most ability to comprehend the issues involved. Competency is not easy to gauge, as it involves a number of judgments: the capacity to reason, the ability to recall, and the ability to comprehend and integrate the information given. There must be freedom from significant psychological influence, such as depression or undue anxiety. In difficult situations, a third person who has special expertise in this area may share in the assessment of competency. The more that healthcare providers can enter into a relationship with the person making the decision, the more that person will be able to participate in a comprehended choice of what should be done.

Shared decision making and consent or comprehended choice is a dynamic, ongoing process. The unfortunate necessity of linking consent so visibly to consent forms, in most institutions, makes it easy to overlook the process that is required to cover each and every contact with the individual each day. This is to say that, even "ordinary" procedures, such as obtaining blood pressure, bathing a patient, or taking a blood sample need consent. In emergencies, comprehended choice should still be obtained, if at all possible. If the medical condition requires immediate attention and time does not permit fully informed or comprehended consent, professionals can act without consent. If the situation is less urgent, but the patient is deemed to lack competency, two physicians, one not directly involved in the case, should concur on a course of action in writing, in addition to informing family members. At all times the person's values, such as those found in a written or verbal advance directive, should, if known, dominate the decision making.

A healthcare provider, when asked to witness a written consent, who doubts that the consenting person fully comprehends the issue or is unsure that the consenting person has been given adequate information to make a comprehended choice, may be obliged by professional ethics to refuse to act as a witness. In law, this point is confusing, since the witness is said only to be witnessing the signature and not the level of a person's understanding. But professional ethical behavior, in such a situation, demands more than compliance with the law. When patients lack competency to make healthcare decisions, they need a substitute decision maker. The mechanism for this prior delegation is an advance directive, a "living will," or the legally recognized equivalent.

Shared decision making is a particularly difficult process when patients have psychiatric or mental disabilities. Persons who need temporary confinement in an institution for their own or for others' safety are not thereby deprived of their civil rights, but may still not agree to what careproviders deem to be appropriate treatment. Newer mental health laws attempt to lay out humane ways, using tribunals and other consultations, to preserve and respect affected persons' dignity and autonomy, as well as their safety. Patients who are restless, easily antagonized, noisy, or violent are vulnerable to abuse through the use of restraints, which may be physical (bodily restraint or segregation, as in isolated confinement), pharmacological, or even psychological (such as when patients are isolated or ignored). Yet such action may be necessary to protect others (staff and other persons) as well as the patients (from themselves). Consultation and continual vigilance (review of restraint) are necessary to navigate through these ethical hazards.

Competent persons who have been adequately informed of the options—the potential benefits and risk—may refuse any or all treatment, and their decisions are binding. Included in the commitment to informed consent is an injunction not to give information to the family that is not also given to the patient. Indeed, a competent person in need should be consulted, and should agree, before the family is given personal information. When there is family conflict, providers will want to assist the family in resolving disagreements by inviting family members to conferences and/or suggesting assistance from various sources (family advisors, religious persons, family friends, or advocates, as well as through ethical consultation). While informed choice focuses on individuals and their ability to make choices, we now want to look more closely at the field of choices that affect and are affected by individuals' choices. We will now turn back to the decision making of Joanna and Paul.

INDIVIDUAL CHOICES

As we follow the story of Paul and Joanna, we will be able to see the impact of their choice on themselves and their relations with Paul's parents, Joanna's doctor, the hospital department, the healthcare system, and the community. By identifying these influences, we will begin to see that each relationship and each decision affects many or perhaps all other relationships. When a stone is thrown into a pond, the ripples touch the whole pond. Although the impact of a decision is greater for those who make the decision, the ripples created by the decision made will extend to those who may not even recognize what it means to them. The environment of a decision is the *whole* of which we, each one of us, are a part. Of course this does not mean that individual autonomy and freedom are not respected. In a way, it's the ultimate respect of autonomy that we share the discussion and we share the decision by the discussion—sorting it out again and again for as long as necessary for people to feel they are satisfied with their own decision. It is a false notion to think that by just having the facts, we can easily make a decision.

As we consider Joanna and Paul's dilemma in making a decision about whether or not to continue with the pregnancy, the complexities are found within the freedom to make ethical decisions in real life. It could be easy to focus on the communication and counseling skills used by the doctor in giving diagnostic information. We could even consider better ways to give difficult news like this to parents.[3] But in this text, we want to focus on the network of relations that affect the freedom and the responsibility of the various individuals to choose. In the video of Joanna and Paul, the responsibility of choice or decision was passed from one to another: The doctor says to the parents, "It's up to you," and the wife says to the husband, "It's up to you." We suggest that there could be a broader way to understand individual choice—individual decision making that is grounded in the web of relation. So whose choice is it?

Is it the parents' choice? As stated above, the concept of informed consent is based on the right of each person to give

consent to anything that is done to that person. Health professionals are compelled by both ethical duty and the law to give
reliable and adequate information to patients so that they may
make choices that are informed. This means that information
about procedures, treatments, and choices is based on each
person's ability to comprehend. In Paul and Joanna's situation, the doctor tried to be perfectly clear about the nature of
the problem. She said, "Of course, the baby would not be able
to walk." But even then she had to qualify her sureness by
saying, "Well, perhaps, someday, with a walker or. . . . " The
doctor was even less sure about the infant's potential cognitive ability. Although it was very clear that the baby had spina
bifida, it was very unclear as to the actual complexity of the
problem. Such uncertainty is always present in real life, and
certainly for parents—any parents. The health of an unborn
child is always a mystery—felt in the space where we, as parents, catch our breath until the baby takes its first breath.[4] The
reality of being a parent is felt in the fear that our baby will be
sick, disabled, hurt, or even die.

Is it the father's choice? Some might expect the father to
make the choice here, because he is seen as responsible to
support his child through its life. The fact that Joanna also
needs assistance may make it seem as though Paul will carry
the burden of the care, and therefore the decision should be
his. When we are on our own, without community or financial support, the burden of care for anyone, each child, one
another, can become an overburden. The word "burden" comes
from the same etymological Indo-European root *bher*, which
also means to bear or to birth children.[5] Having children, having a child, is always a burden—a fact pointed out by Joanna.
There are risks and burdens with birthing children. Some of
us have come to believe that having children with special
needs can be more of a burden than parents or society is willing to bear. We have seen parents overburdened by care of
children born with severe medical problems without the support and sustenance of a committed community. Of course,
fathers need to be decision makers. Fathers need to commit
themselves to the life-long burden of caring for their children.
Because fathers do not have the embodied experience of preg-

nancy—of carrying a developing child within their own body—they have to make the commitment to the child in a different way than women do. They have to consciously and deliberately say "yes" to a child as their own. While the father must decide, he does so without any effect on his bodily integrity. His decision comes from a different experience than that of the mother.

Is it the mother's choice? Termination of a pregnancy involves the mother, so we need to ensure that the mother would be a decision maker. The mother would definitely need to consent to any decision to terminate the pregnancy. She must comprehend what this decision will mean to her. As the mother, she is already experiencing the reality of the baby, with her changed physical body and perhaps even feeling the movement of the baby. Technology, however, gives information about the baby that she cannot experience in her body. While her body is already saying "yes" to this pregnancy as it grows and changes, the use of a prenatal diagnosis procedure results in the mother's tentativeness in responding to the growing baby—she has to hold herself back from engaging too closely with her growing child.[6] Through technology, the mother is given information that forces another choice on her. Her decision now is to say "no" to this pregnancy and this potential child. When a mother says "no," she is bodily involved.

Yet we begin to see how complicated such a decision is for this mother, for Joanna. It is not just a decision about understanding the procedure and its personal and medical and surgical risks for her. It is not just about her decision of whether or not she will let go of this pregnancy and perhaps "try again." In making a decision to terminate this pregnancy because of spina bifida, Joanna also comes to question the value and meaning of her own life. In the video, Joanna says something like, "If we abort this child we might be suggesting that my life is meaningless. I shouldn't be here. My mother should have aborted me." If she refuses to birth the child because of spina bifida, does she not also ask herself, "Should I have been born?" or "Am I valid?" The mother's choice then is not one based merely on the facts—the potential for the baby to walk, for example. Not only is the mother asked to make a decision about whether or not to terminate her pregnancy, she is also forced, unexpectedly perhaps, to face the worth of her own life—to herself, to her family, and to her community. She is forced to question her relationships and how these relationships are value-laden. Her identity is tied to others through the network of relationships—the value that others give to her life. It becomes clear that it is the mother's choice, yet the impact of her choice is not just on her alone; the community is affected. Relationships are affected.

Is it the baby's choice? How could we possibly think about the baby having any part in this decision? Perhaps a better question is, How does the baby influence the mother's or the parents' choice? Finding out that the child is a girl—not an "it"—seems to make a difference for Joanna. It seems that, as the mother comes to relate to the child, as a girl and as a daughter, her freedom to choose changes. Could this relational connection make any difference to Joanna in coming to her decision? Should she even have been told the sex of the fetus? If not, why not? If she does decide to terminate the pregnancy with this changed reality, will Joanna grieve her loss differently—as a lost child rather than a lost pregnancy? Is there a difference?

A discussion occurred in the research group that adds another dimension to considering about how decisions are made. Here we began to question whether rational and factual considerations are the only ones available to humans.

I'm struck by the similarity to the discussion we had when we looked at A Choice for K'aila [see chapter three] *and about a concept that just intrigued me at that time and continues to intrigue me. I think you called it* mutual thinking. *There is a kind of way in which people experience coming to decision from different points of view. That's what K'aila's mom had experienced. Have I captured it? . . .*

Yes. And it's not my concept, you know. It's a concept in Cree cosmology and it is that collective decision making is better than just the individual—there's more power to it. There's more authenticity to it and there are pro-

cesses that involve not just talking about it. It is about understanding together. It's the kind of thinking that goes on silently around a fire so, you know, that understanding, that unspoken focus and then everybody knows what's to be done. I don't think White people have the concept. That's why it's hard to articulate. . . .

To think mutually with someone else, though, you have to respect his or her autonomy. You can't have mutual thinking without that mutual respect. That's one of the things in the video you see. You look at the miscommunications between the two of them [Joanna and Paul] because tacit in all of that discussion is what she articulated about the value of her life.[7]

The discussion illustrated here points to the quality of our humanness, the quality that gets mutilated when we make an arbitrary distinction between feeling and reason.[8] In the above discussion, we recognized that rationality is broader than merely thinking—that there is more to "account for" than the words. In real talk we do not exchange information in a mechanistic way, like computers. There are, of course, aspects of communication that encompass a particular skill, but they are just a mere part of the discourse. Rather, there is something that happens "between the words," or in the "way" one speaks. Within the concept of mutual thinking, communication is physical, emotional, cognitive, and spiritual, all at once. The concept of mutual thinking is concerned with the embodied connection—not just the words, but the personhood of the person with whom we interact. Mutual thinking is talking *with* others, not *to* others, and is a process through which "meeting of the minds" is a result. Of course, not all encounters involve mutual thinking; rather, there are "flashes"—those times when we have been discussing something with others and we realize that we have the same (roughly at the same time) idea or thought.

In order to understand choice and decision-making issues in the magnitude of life and death, we need to consider that knowledge and understanding includes the body and spirit as well as the mind. With Joanna's connection to her unborn child, she understands the wholeness of her child, herself, and her community—the mutual fragility of life, the reflection on the value of her own life, and the possibilities presented in any child's life.

SOCIETAL CHOICES

Is this choice society's to make? What role do societal attitudes and perspectives have to play in individual decision making? We're facing decisions now, in genetics, about what kinds of humans we will accept in our community and what value we give people who are different. How do we accept difference? How do we value difference? And, underlying these questions, is our question about what is "normal." It is not hard to recognize the different opinions communities have about choices that Joanna and Paul are facing. Some feel that every stage of human life—including embryo and fetus—demands a right to life, regardless of its actual or potential attributes. Others feel that now that we have the technical ability to screen for severe disabling conditions, we have no right to bring children with severe problems into the world. A newspaper letter to the editor of the Toronto *Globe and Mail* demonstrates the extent and passion of public opinion. The letter condemns parents' decision to knowingly continue a pregnancy and give birth to a disabled child. "This was, first of all, not fair to Francine [the disabled child], who has to suffer the consequences of that decision for the rest of her life. It was not fair to her brother, who will now take second place when it comes to getting attention. It certainly is not fair to the rest of society, which is now expected to assist the family even though the situation could have been avoided."[9]

Others have described the blessings experienced through the care of their disabled children.[10] In describing her relationship with her severely disabled 30-year-old daughter, Eva Feder Kittay says, "For my daughter, dependence of the most profound sort will be part of her 'normal' existence. But such dependence does not preclude a certain form of mutual dependence. I depend on her as well. Sesha and her well-being are essential to my own. . . . Watching her grow and develop skills and take pride in her accomplishments nurtures me as much as my own work."[11] Here, Kittay, a mother and scholar, acknowledges that it was a moment of discovery to recognize that while her daughter is completely dependent on her and others, Kittay, herself, as a person, depends on her daughter in significant ways. Jean Vanier, in the published Massey Lecture Series, suggests that, through openness to weakness, to being different, or even to being inferior, is how we achieve personal and societal freedom.[12] "If we deny our weakness and the reality of death, if we want to be powerful and strong always, we deny a part of our being, we live in illusion. To be human is to accept who we are, this mixture of strength and weakness."[13]

When we consider choice and decision, we right away are caught in an environment that supports or encourages certain choices over other choices. The choice and decision making, the signing of the consent form, falls to one person, or one set of parents, yet all of us, as environment, are implicated. The decision that Paul and Joanna make affects us. Will society welcome a child born with spina bifida? Will society be willing to share resources in the care for this child? Every time we make an individual decision in a society, we're not only making a decision (especially on something like prenatal diagnosis) just for ourselves, but also a decision that affects others. However much we hold individual freedom as expressed in personal choice, each choice does affect others. We are a society as a whole.

The disability and ethics literature outlines two primary models of community attitudes toward disability. The *biomedical model* focuses on the medical condition or personal attribute (on the ability to walk, see, hear, or on cognition) as a limitation that needs medical intervention. *The social model* focuses on the individual condition (on the ability to walk, and so forth) as limitations only because of socially constructed barriers. Within the biomedical model, attention is focused on assessing, preventing, treating, or ameliorating the disability of the individual. The biomedical model views a disability as a problem to be prevented or repaired through medical technology. Within this model, the person who is disabled is often seen as a patient who needs to be "fixed" or "treated." Sometimes the disabled person is looked upon with pity or rejection. Ideological reduction is one obvious fear created by the extremes of a biomedical model, because it can lead to the atrocities of genocide.[14] The biomedical model is an individualistic model that can be extended ideologically to include groups or even races. The social model presents disability as a socially created problem, and we must come to understand that it is society that creates disability. We are only lately prepared to give as much community support to providing ramps for wheelchairs as we are for cars and trucks. It is each of us that create the environment where everyone, of whatever ability, is able to flourish to the extent of our ability. The social model does not speak about patients or to the specific attributes of a person's body or mind, but looks to how the person participates and is integrated into community life. The social model is a collective or interactive model. As Gregor Wolbring notes, it shows the collective responsibility to create an environment "for the full participation of people with different biological realities in all areas of social life. . . . The social model allows 'able-ism' to be seen in the same light as racism or sexism."[15]

FREEDOM AND WHOLENESS

Both the social and biomedical models have value, and both have limitations. We as individuals desire—indeed expect—that the healthcare system will provide us with all services that will enable us to hear better, to see better, to walk more easily, or to think more ably—that is, to be "fixed." At the same time, we want to have the services and attitudes that attend the social model, which enhances our ability to live as fulfilling a life as possible. Perhaps the real danger of either model is to again get caught in the dualism of either/or—which then becomes a battle of models. Distinctions are useful in clarifying the issues that are at stake, but instead of being silent or taking sides,[16] what might be most helpful is to hold the tension of both models in a relational space so that new understandings can develop. The time has come, says Erich Neumann, for "the principle of perfection to be sacrificed on the altar of wholeness."[17] According to Neumann, wholeness occurs when we accept the actual state of imperfection—personal and societal limitations (weaknesses, personal shadows, evils) as well as strengths. Wholeness, not perfection or happiness, is the goal that integrates all parts of ourselves, not placing or "scapegoating" the negative on others, whether of a different race, religion, gender, ableness, or goodness. Wholeness is not limited by a person's ability to walk or to see.

Wholeness lives with the tension felt by the incorporation or integration of the opposites—the weak in the strong, the able in the disabled, the evil in the good. It is not so hard to imagine "perfection" sacrificed for "wholeness" when we observe athletes with varying abilities (for example, whether racing on legs or in wheelchairs) strive for personal and national best. It is harder to imagine perfection sacrificed to wholeness when we think of extremely painful, limiting conditions— whether they come with birth or injury. It is even harder to think of wholeness when integrating and accepting both good and evil, happiness and suffering within each of us—not holding "us" as good and "others" as evil. But the space for wholeness is more than just within the individual. Wholeness integrates the individual within the collective, the bigger world. Wholeness, which holds the tension of both the biomedical and social model, could lead to genuine respect for other people, other groups, other abilities, and other forms and levels of culture,[18] because it respects the otherness (weakness, illness, shadow, unconscious, evil) within ourselves as well. With wholeness, there is room for dependence as well as independence. Attention to wholeness may also mean that resources and services are available to alleviate suffering and limitation. Attention to wholeness integrates biomedical and social models by a focus of interdependence rather than independence. In fact, attention to wholeness values diversity and creates a place for understanding and support, rather than division and isolation.

The relational ethic is a web, and the major feature of this web is *interdependence* (which holds dependence and independence equally valuable). Interdependence is the relationship of being true to ourselves and open to the other, committed to ourselves as individuals as well as ourselves as environment—connections between people, institutions, agencies, and other structures. By attending to interdependence, we are also brought to attention of the true autonomy of each—but this autonomy is not one-sided and individualistic, but integrated into the needs and commitments of the society. Based on the work of John Macmurray, Enrique Dussel, and others, we have come to understand that the freedom of any person is bound up and dependent on the freedom and integrity of all.[19] Freedom is achieved through interdependence, for interdependence expects reciprocity. Freedom can only be achieved through reciprocal interdependence.[20] As James Olthuis says, freedom "begins with a recognition of difference—not as deviance or deficit that threatens—but as otherness to connect with, cherish, and celebrate."[21] As we connect with difference—as Dussel notes, not as a "mere *difference* but as the truly *distinct*, as wholly Other"[22]—we find wholeness. In wholeness we can let go of both happiness and guilt, and in doing so we can find a new consciousness, what Erich Neumann calls a new morality—not surrendering to disease, weakness, or even evil or projecting it on someone else,[23] but accepting difference within oneself and within the other. "Accepting and recognizing differences is a process fraught with apprehension and anxiety, either working together towards a community-in-difference (where justice and compassion flourish) or a falling apart into islands of opposition (and the spread of rancor and hate)."[24] *This* is our choice.

UNCERTAINTY'S TRUTH

One of the consistent concerns about a move away from a purely normative ethics is that it will become so diluted that it slips into moral relativism, nihilism, or chaos.[25] While we propose that relational ethics cannot be reduced to principles, we contend that it is not relativistic and will not lead to chaos. It is held together by the recognition of our mutual interdependence. It is also held by the possibility of sustaining a humane world where we can come together as community. Being governed by laws, rules, and principles is not enough, because this reduces us to dualities. Rather, relationship is important primarily because, through relational space, we can integrate and grow. Relational space is not an entity by itself, but only exists through connection between people. Relational space holds individuals and groups together. To reject the pursuit of absolutes—sureness or perfection—does not mean that all avenues of action are perceived as being equal. There are still decisions to be made—for example, there remain pregnancies that, for complex reasons, might be terminated.

In taking the practice of ethical thinking into how we can make our relationships flourish, we place increasing emphasis on the question rather than the answer, on uncertainty rather than sureness, and on the integrity that is found in the middle. Uncertainty is a truth that asks for humility rather than power, understanding rather than information, and relationship rather than ideology. By bringing us back to the relational space of healthcare practice, we recognize that power, of course, is present. Power held in this ethical place is less sure of itself. By creating this "between" space, there is room for considering numerous possibilities. Relational space is an ambiguous space where certainty does not exist. Our challenge is living and being comfortable with ambiguity—not only in searching for control.

In searching for understanding in place of the control that ideologies and rules hope to bring, we suggest the notion of a middle ground that cautions us against taking any stance (knowingly or unknowingly) that says "my truth is the only truth." Sometimes patients take this controlling stance, sometimes the caregivers; sometimes it is a religion, sometimes a national consensus; or sometimes it is an ethical expert or the law. In these situations, it may be that ideology gets mistaken for the truth, as ideology's great moral shortcoming is its failure to see the bigger picture. The opposite of this view is equally unacceptable and untrue—where abject relativeness sees moral value, knowledge, or truth relative to individual, historical circumstances or culture. But the middle ground, or relational space, is not "relative"—it is enclosed by mutual respect, engagement, embodiment, and dialogue. It recognizes the truth of relationship—a truth that finds that our choices affect both you and me. The wonderful, ever-shifting, ambiguous middle ground is a place that is approached with humility, knowing that we—none of us—have the whole picture, the Truth with a capital "T." There is a recognition that we cannot see the whole picture. Such recognition asks for humility.

Particularity is the key—the need for cultural traditions, seeing the truths there; the need for old morals and old gods, and seeing truths there. Particularity is the key because it grounds us in practical life. The particular stories of K'aila, Dax, Allison, and Paul and Joanna call attention to the middle ground. This middle ground is not the place to find the Solution with a capital "S." Instead, it may be possible to find smaller solutions—myriad small solutions along the way. These solutions are not primarily actions taken after a problem-solving exercise that has, as its goal, to be problem-free. Instead, these solutions result in understanding the dilemma that is faced by each individual—giving it depth and value, giving it expression and meaning. As Raimond Gaita notes, "If we are wise we will not want to settle dilemmas too quickly by someone who takes it to be relatively clear, or by someone who thinks relatively quickly that they know what the issues mean to each of the participants."[26] The middle ground, a creative place, is a place where ethical issues can never be resolved with absolute certainty. Rather, in such a place, the issues become more complex. In such a place, we need to know the personal story as well as to have normative knowledge. In such a place, we need to open our hearts to blending the highest understanding of subjectivity with the highest understanding of objectivity.[27]

ENVIRONMENT AS WHOLENESS

We have proposed that each individual choice affects other choices. Each transplantation decision affects all the other people who wait for a transplant. Each decision to terminate a pregnancy because of disability does affect attitudes toward disability. All children who are born, no matter if cognitively gifted or cognitively impaired, call on social and political will to create room for them in community. We live in one world. Such an acknowledgment accepts the fact that what we as people do in our homes, hospitals, laboratories, doctors' offices, cities, nations, does affect others in other places and times. We live in one world, one globe, where breathe the same air! With John Donne's famous line, "No man is an island, entire of itself; every man is a piece of the continent, a part of the man," we feel the interconnected and interdependent world we live in where, "any man's death diminishes me, because I am involved in mankind, and therefore never send to know for whom the bell tolls; it tolls for thee." [28]

In our human community, we recognize that there is a link between respect for individual autonomy and the responsibility of autonomy for other individuals and for society as a whole. The strong focus on autonomy and human rights in bioethics has sometimes eclipsed issues of social justice—attention to an interconnected community. While it would be completely inappropriate to give up on autonomy, there is a danger that autonomy can become a thin notion when we do not give equal attention to the relationship in which autonomy is fostered. It might be helpful to think of the distinction between an autonomous person and a person who lives from their own authority, suggested by Polly Young-Eisendrath and Florence Wiedemann. They describe autonomous persons as those who act only from their own will, with little concern for the values or needs of others; they decribe persons who act from a place of "personal authorship" as authors of their own lives, who respond flexibly and reciprocally to a variety of desires and needs that come from both the self and from others. [29] Personal authorship suggests an interactive process; persons who know their own autonomy and their own values may respond empathetically and decisively to each new situation within a network of relations. Being for, and with, others does not mean that we lose ourselves. In some situations, the focus of individual autonomy has undermined the concept of community, and this lack of attention to community has been detrimental to society as a whole, and to many of its citizens.

EARTH AS COMMUNITY

So far in this chapter we have focused on the interdependence between individual persons and the community in making informed choices, but, as we explore relationships, we cannot stop there. We need to consider the biophysical sphere as well. The fact that we all breathe the same air re-

minds us that if we describe community as only relations between people, we still fall short. What seems to be required
from us now is a larger recognition—the recognition of the
earth as our community. The earth is our community. As Larry
Rasmussen writes, "Earth—all of it—is a community without
an exit. Our problems—people-to-people and humankind-to-
otherkind—are genuinely ours all together, for worse or for
better."[30] If we commit to the reality that the earth is our community, then we recognize that the environment is not something "out there" to which we have a responsibility. Environment means the place we are "in," right now, right here. We—
the public, professionals, patients, families, administrators,
the government, the world—are *the* healthcare system. There
is no vantage point from which we can see the world outside
of ourselves—we are in the midst of the world.

Yet to say we all are the environment does not give proper
place to the incredible importance of every small moment of
how we enter relationship with our patients, how we relate to
our colleagues, how we set economic priorities, and what we
expect from ourselves, others, and the earth. Each small moment builds on each other. This book focuses attention on
relations with one another, which, as Rasmussen says, is a
practicality that is tied to the "great new fact of our time, which
is that cumulative human activity has the power to affect all
life in fundamental and unprecedented ways."[31] The question that we have asked throughout this text, *How ought we to
live?* takes on even more significance when we apprehend
Rassmussen's view of our "fundamentally changed human relationship to the earth, a relationship we only partially comprehend."[32] These relations are built in the places where we
live (cities, towns, countries), the places where we work (hospitals, clinics, agencies, and institutions), the lands we love
(countries and nations), the one world (earth), and the many
galaxies that hold the earth in place. When we think of healthcare ethics, we often forget our primal ethic: recognition of
the place (the earth) we are in and our responsibility for it.

A relational ethic speaks to relationships between us, all
of us, whether or whenever we are professionals or patients,
providers or receivers; whatever race, gender, ableness, or age
we are; whether rich or poor, strong or weak, saints or sin-

ners. And the relations between us are deeply affected by and affect our relationship to our world, the earth, and its creatures—all of them. Our diversity is not limited to the color of our skin, the food we eat, the songs we sing. Rather, our diversity is most vividly experienced in our attitudes toward ourselves, each other, other creatures, and our world. Our differing opinions, beliefs, and religions vividly show a diversity that may not always be easy to accept. Some of us are fascinated by genetic mapping, others of us are fearful that such mapping will result in humans being identified only by our genes; some value the potential of choosing one's child's characteristics, others fear that such choices lead to intolerance; some value the ability to do anything that is possible in research and technology and others fear the loss of compassion and meaningfulness of life. Many fear that commodification of life will be the death of life. Yes, the ethical challenges are immense, and our commitment to embrace these challenges must also be immense. Where is commitment found? Our commitments to the world, and to each other, are experienced through close relationships—to each other and to the earth.

We live in a world in which social bonds seem to be disintegrating, in which violent actions are mutually destructive (hurting both the violated and the violator), and in which extreme disparities occur, not just between the wealthy and the poor, but the excessively rich (beyond all need) and the excessively poor (beyond all description). We know that there are also great disparities in health and healthcare; in some places in the world (such as Canada and the United States) people with HIV/AIDS receive drugs and services, while in other places (such as Africa) thousands of people die daily from want of the same drugs and services. Stephen Lewis, the United Nations' Special Envoy for HIV/AIDS in Africa, suggests that Western nations let this happen through complacency.[33]

Has apathy become the norm in issues of morality? Even with the taken-for-granted activities like transplants—skin, hearts, and kidneys—do we need caution? With the possibility of face transplants, it is not so foolish to be concerned, as Rasmussen notes, that the skin we transplant is both healthy and sensitive—for skin needs to be sensitive in order to respond.[34] While transplanted hearts need to have a chemical makeup that will be accepted by the new body, hearts also need to be tender! We want skin and hearts that are sensitive to the pain of the world and to each other. Our ethical response is lost when our skin becomes callused and unfeeling, or when our hearts become only biological parts. Should this happen, we will become disinterested and indifferent. But we still have a chance. We are still moved by pain. Pain leaves us with an aching heart, and while no one wants an aching heart, as Rasmussen notes, "it is preferable to an empty one."[35]

Let us think for a moment about the rapidly developing world of transplantation. What does transplantation practice do to our relationships? Imagine the poignancy of walking around with someone else's bone marrow or kidney. Surely there are few bonds that are stronger than between a donor family, who has lost a loved one, and the person who receives a vital organ, so life itself remains. While there are good reasons, such as the risk of exploitation, for strict confidentiality on specifics between donors and recipients, there may also be a true bridge to community solidarity here as well. The potential of these bonds is seen through the increasing number of memorial days and donor family recognition events. Could transplantation be the example that builds community and our commitment to well-being of each other?

The crisis in the environment is a crisis of culture, the nature of community. The sense of the whole is to see that the healthcare system is really just another system. Such a system, says David Seedhouse, can be changed by using the way of culture, "to work in a partly logical, partly emotional fashion in a way that acknowledges history and culture."[36] With violent and disastrous conflicts erupting all around the world, with economic disparities growing larger, with the piling on of more and more knowledge sent rapidly around the world, we feel the lack of a whole. Yet we need the wholeness of a sustainable community with an eye to human responsibility and self-understanding. We need to consider the view of a single interconnected civilization; as Rasmussen says, "a common story to live by."[37] We need to consider the little, everyday actions that make a difference to the big picture. Individual moments—moral actions—can become movements. As

Rasmussen notes, "Indeed, moral formation of society and world is a critical *action* of its own—or, rather, a million small actions undertaken by everyone."[38] If we do need one standard to live by, perhaps we should consider Walter Jeffko's community standard, which "refers to the good and well-being—what Macmurray calls the 'harmony'—of each and every person in both relational and individual aspects."[39] In his clarification, Jeffko reminds us that it is not only how we treat others but "how one treats oneself [that] has moral significance."[40] Jeffko outlines the minimal elements of a principle of community: (1) the person must be treated as a whole, not merely a function or characteristic, (2) love is the motive of the relation, (3) equality must be present if the relation is interpersonal, and (4) we treat each other with as much freedom as the relation will allow.[41] While Jeffko uses friendship as the ideal personal relation that holds the community standard, he argues that there are other relations that offer examples: the teacher-student, and, we suggest, the healthcare professional and patient and family. The community standard, from a relational ethic viewpoint, bridges the gap between the duality of the traditional Kantian ethics of justice and equality and the care ethic of love and compassion.[42] The community standard transcends the opposition of justice and care. We propose that a *principle of community* would need to extend to the larger world—our environment. Gabriel Marcel, in 1943, wrote of the need for moral renewal, which would involve "small communities coming together like swarms one after the other" to form what he called centers of example, which would be "nuclei of life around which the lacerated tissues of true moral existence can be reconstituted."[43] Perhaps we can again look for examples of how we can learn how to live together, in spite of our diversities and difference.

CENTERS OF EXAMPLE

If our ethical interest is in the *quality of our relationships,* then intersubjectivity or interconnectedness will be given our first attention. Facing the reality of our interconnectedness brings us face-to-face with "difference." We live in a world where differences are more and more evident, and with attention to difference we become more aware of inequalities and partialities. With intersubjectivity as our goal, rather than valuing models of control, in which emphasis is given to *power-over* or *freedom-from*, we will look for models that advocate *power-with* and *freedom-to*, and in which individual identity and empowerment are generated, nourished, and enriched. We will now present two examples that search for change through a focus on the quality of relationships:[44] James Olthuis's research on families,[45] and the experience of two cultures (Jews and Palestinian Arabs of Israeli citizenship) living and working together.[46]

Through research into the relevant correlation between family forms and levels of violence, Olthuis and his colleague Catherine Crawford Thompson[47] found that there was a need to rethink the philosophy of the family. By individual interviews with street youth, and through focused discussions with groups of youth, Olthuis and Thompson found young people listed *listening, understanding,* and *assurance of worth* as the top three unmet needs within their families. These young people said they were living on the street "because they had not been welcomed, recognized, embraced, blessed, or shown mercy" within their families.[48] This research challenges standard theories, in which families are discussed in terms of function, role, or type, and proposes that what is really at stake is the presence or lack of intimate connecting. Olthius writes, "Being cared for within the family, we experience belonging, trust, empowerment, connection—and learn to be at ease in the world. It is in the family that compassion begins to root in our souls."[49] He suggests that speaking about families in terms of functional effectiveness or dysfunction dehumanizes the reality of pain, darkness, and suffering those families experience. Violence, he says, whether in families or nations, has to do with the "lost world of feelings."[50] Again, Olthuis points to the quality of relationship, and reminds us that healing and recovery do not occur in isolation, but rather happen best in relationships in which compassion, rather than judgment, is needed.

As we begin the twenty-first century, we find ourselves in a world of great disparities and clashes between cultures, ideologies, and religions. Violence and killing are escalating in many places around the world. A small intentional community, Neve Shalom/Wahat al Salam (NSWAS), situated equidistant from Jerusalem and Tel Aviv-Jaffa, may be another kind of example that can move us from the moment to a movement.[51] This cooperative village of Jews and Palestinian Arabs of Israeli citizenship, begun in the early 1970s, demonstrates the possibility of co-existence of these two divergent and historically hostile groups. The intention of this community is mutual acceptance, respect, and cooperation. The village has a number of activities that foster and develop its vision, primarily through education, and there is equal participation by children, youth, and adults from both groups. This small community began with a school in which only the village children participated, but now educational activities are open to children from outside the village as well. The children learn about their own identity, culture, and traditions, and at the same time learn to accept and appreciate each other. The village also sponsors the School of Peace, which conducts outreach work informed by a vision of a humane, egalitarian, and just society that will evolve out of students' interaction with each other. These educational sessions, in which both Hebrew and Arabic languages are used, provide conflict resolution opportunities with empowerment of Arab and Jewish women, as well as men, as one of the goals. The village also has a center for spiritual pluralism, where people of all creeds and cultures can reflect through meditation and prayer. The House of Silence is a place for reflection and research in the role of spiritual and ethical values for the advancement of peace. Although the NSWAS or Oasis for Peace is just a small community—just a moment in the bigger world—its vision has the potential to spread. NSWAS was one of two recipients of the 2002 annual award by UNICEF that conducts work aiming to produce a better future for children. "It is always risky to be lured by metaphors, especially in the Middle East," says Anton Shammas, a Palestinian writer, "but those who live in this 'Oasis of Peace' have managed to achieve the impossible: by refusing to be lured, they have concretized a methaphor. We, who are still wandering in the desert, envy them."[52] Can we learn from them as well?

These examples are initiatives in which the intention is to build understanding through working together with people who come from different backgrounds, communities, ideologies, race, history, experience, and scholarship. The intent is to create opportunities for understanding, sharing of ideas, hearing different points of view, and valuing all points of view as worthy of attention that will lead to greater responsibility for all. We are at a time, are we not, when recognizing our common humanity needs to override the religious ideologies and history that keep us apart?

CONCLUSION

We do not learn from the video *Who Should Decide?* what decision Joanna and Paul make in relation to the findings of prenatal diagnosis. Whatever their decision, the goal would be that they would be able to consider a broad range of choices through exploring all aspects of the situation—to be able to make a comprehended choice. They may decide to terminate the pregnancy and "try again" to conceive a child without spina bifida. This would fit most closely with the current expectation that we should bring the healthiest babies into the world. They might decide to maintain the pregnancy and prepare themselves for the birth of a baby with spina bifida without knowing what it would be like for them as parents. This decision would be more in line with the belief that all children, of whatever capability, have a right to life, family, and a community that provides opportunities for all children to live happily and well. Whatever their decision, it does affect each of us—in ways that are subtle rather than overt, that are supportive of our own approach or not, but deserve consideration and respect. The move to wholeness that we have been exploring in this chapter finds support in the words of a young woman, Karyn Christensen, who is going blind, who says, "Whether there is stereotypical notion of norm or not, we all work at providing safety, security, and quality of life for those around us and ourselves. We all contribute to the whole. I believe, there is not a normal or abnormal, just different. Meeting the special needs of the less able requires thought and

sensitivity. Understanding our differences, we can adapt together to sustain quality of life for everyone."[53]

We know the challenges of the healthcare world; we have
heard the voices of Dax, K'aila's mother, Allison's family, and
Joanna and Paul. In each of these stories, we sense the concern for the environment—the family network, the healthcare
system, community expectations, the law, and the courts. Do
we have enough time to be engaged with each other? Do we
have time and energy to contemplate what should be done—
not just what can be done? The ethical questions *What should
I do? What should I know?* are living questions, questions that
are dynamic, ongoing, and exciting. The challenges are immense, and the rewards are also immense.

The poet Olive Schreiner, in 1890, wrote about the gifts of
both freedom and love that were presented to a dreamer as
she slept.[54] In the dream, Life held a gift in each hand—in the
one Love, in the other Freedom. Life asked the dreamer to
choose Love or Freedom. After a long pause, the dreamer chose
Freedom. Life indicated that the dreamer had chosen well,
for with Freedom, Love would be possible as well. Life needed
both Freedom and Love, or Life itself would die. Now, over a
hundred years later, Schreiner's message is still relevant—in
healthcare ethics, as in life, we need both freedom and love.
We need the individual freedom to make decisions and choices
for ourselves, and we need love and compassion for others as
well. The philosopher Luce Irigaray, in 2002, asked why the
wisdom of love has been forgotten, and proposed that the
meaning of philosophy include both the wisdom of love as
well as the love of wisdom (the traditional meaning of philosophy).[55] According to Irigaray, "This possible interpretation would imply that philosophy joins together, more than it
has done in the West, the body, the heart, and the mind. . . . It
would be less a normative science of the truth than the search
for measures that help in living better: with oneself, with others, with the world."[56] Irigaray calls us to a discourse, "a different discourse, a different logic, a different relation to perfection . . . into the elaboration of a shared universe."[57]

Perhaps Schreiner and Irigaray both point in the same direction. Perhaps this is the time to take up both gifts—love as

well as freedom; the wisdom of love and the love of wisdom. If freedom and wisdom are the only gifts of life, without the temperance of love, there is danger of loss of life itself. We propose that we need attention to the autonomous freedom of the individual within an environment of love, compassion, and community with others with whom we share this world.

NOTES

1. Solomon R. Benatar, "Just Healthcare Beyond Individualism: Challenges for North American Bioethics," *Cambridge Quarterly of Healthcare Ethics* 6, no. 4 (1997): 397-415, 398; see also Wendy Austin, "Nursing Ethics in an Era of Globalization," *Advances in Nursing Science* 24, no. 2 (2001): 1-18.
2. *Who Should Decide?* VHS, Discussions in Bioethics Series (Montreal, P.Q.: Centre for Bioethics, Clinical Research Institute Montreal, 1985).
3. Paul Byrne, "Relational Ethics: Giving and Receiving Bad News Following Prenatal Ultrasound Examination," (unpublished research study funded by the Social Sciences and Humanities Research Council of Canada).
4. Vangie Bergum, *A Child on Her Mind: The Experience of Becoming a Mother* (Westport, Conn.: Bergin & Garvey, 1997).
5. William Morris, ed., *The American Heritage Dictionary of the Ethics Language* (Boston: Houghton Mifflin, 1978), 1509.
6. Barbara Katz Rothman, *The Tentative Pregnancy: Prenatal Diagnosis and the Future of Motherhood* (New York: Viking, 1986).
7. Interdisciplinary Research Group #8.
8. Gabriel Marcel, *Home Viator: Introduction to a Metaphysic of Hope,* trans. Emma Craufurd (Gloucester, Mass.: Peter Smith, 1978).
9. Fred Vinzenz, "Letter to the Editor," Toronto *Globe and Mail,* Toronto, Ont.: 20 February 2002, A16.
10. Jean Vanier, *Becoming Human* (Toronto, Ont.: Anansi, 1998); Eva Feder Kittay, "When Caring is Just and Justice is Caring: Justice and Mental Retardation," (paper presented at Feminist Bioethics Association Conference, London, September 2000).
11. Kittay, "When Caring is Just," see note 10 above.
12. Vanier, *Becoming Human,* see note 10 above.
13. Ibid., 40.

14. See Marta Munzarová, "Towards the Abolition of Man: The Voice of Disabled Persons Cannot be Ignored," *Bulletin of Medical Ethics* 174 (2002): 13-21; *Gattaca,* directed by Andrew Niccol (Culver City, Calif.: Columbia Tristar Interactive, 1997).

15. Gregor Wolbring, "Bioethics and Disability: Making Assumptions Explicit," *Health Ethics Today* 12, no. 1 (2001): 17-8.

16. Munzarová, "Towards the Abolition," see note 14 above, p 13.

17. Erich Neumann, *Depth Psychology and a New Ethic,* trans. Eugene Rolfe (New York: G. P. Putnam's Sons, 1969), 134.

18. Ibid., 97.

19. Enrique Dussel, *The Underside of Modernity: APEL, Ricoeur, Rorty, Taylor, and the Philosophy of Liberation,* trans. Eduardo Mendieta (Atlantic Highlands, N.J.: Humanities Press, 1996); John Macmurray, *Persons in Relation,* vol. 2, *The Form of the Personal* (London, U.K.: Faber & Faber, 1961).

20. Mary Ann Bendfeld, "The Limits of Freedom: John Macmurray and Michel Foucault," (unpublished paper, University of Alberta, Edmonton, 1999).

21. James H. Olthuis, ed., *Towards an Ethics of Community: Negotiations of Difference in a Pluralist Society* (Waterloo, Ont.: Wilfrid Laurier University Press, 2000).

22. Dussel, *The Underside of Modernity,* see note 19 above, xvi.

23. See note 17 above, p. 143.

24. See note 21 above, pp. 5-6.

25. Edmund D. Pellegrino, "Bioethics at Century's Turn: Can Normative Ethics Be Retrieved?" *Journal of Medicine and Philosophy* 25, no. 6 (2000): 655-75; Daniel Callahan, "Judging the Future: Whose Fault Will It Be?" *Journal of Medicine and Philosophy* 25, no. 6 (2000): 677-87.

26. Raimond Gaita, *Good and Evil: An Absolute Conception* (London, Macmillan Press, 1991), 127.

27. Polly Young-Eisendrath and Florence L. Wiedemann, *Female Authority* (New York, Guilford Press, 1987).

28. John Donne (1572-1631). *John Donne's Devotions, XVII Meditation* (Grand Rapids, Mich.: Christian Classics Ethereal Library), *http//www.ccel/donne/devotions.ccel.html#1.*

29. See note 27 above.

30. Larry L. Rasmussen, *Earth Community, Earth Ethics* (Maryknoll, N.Y.: Orbis, 1996), xii.

31. Ibid., 5.

32. Ibid.

33. Jonathan Gatehouse. "Crusade for Life. Tribute to Stephen Lewis as Canadian of the Year," [Toronto] *Macleans,* 29 December 2003, p. 20-21.

34. Mary Wollstonecraft wrote in 1792, "Those who are able to see pain, unmoved, will soon learn to inflict it," cited in Rasmussen, see note 30 above, 344.

35. See note 30 above, p. 345.

36. David Seedhouse, cited in Benatar, see note 1 above, p. 406.

37. See note 30 above, p. 16.

38. Ibid., 344.

39. Walter G. Jeffko, *Contemporary Ethical Issues. A Personalistic Perspective* (Amherst, N.Y.: Humanity Books, 1999), 21.

40. Ibid., 22

41. Ibid., 25-26.

42. Ibid., 27.

43. See note 8 above, p. 164.

44. See Vangie Bergum, "Ethical Challenges of the 21st Century: Attending to Relations," *Canadian Journal of Nursing Research* 34, no. 2, 9-15, for earlier discussion of ideas developed here.

45. See note 21 above.

46. Neve Shalom/Wahat al Salam, *http://nswas.com.*

47. Catherine Crawford Thompson, *Reading between the Lines: No Place, No Comfort, No Honor* (Toronto, Ont.: World Vision Canada, 1994).

48. See note 21 above, p. 128.

49. Ibid., 135.

50. Ibid., 138.

51. See note 46 above.

52. See note 46 above, from "What others say about Neve Shalom~Wahat al-Salam."

53. Karyn Christensen, "In the First Person," *Health Ethics Today* 12, no. 1 (2001): 16.

54. Olive Schreiner, *Dreams* (London: Unwin, 1890), 99-100.

55. Luce Irigaray, *The Way of Love* (London, U.K.: Continuum, 2002).

56. Ibid., 2.

57. Ibid., 9.

7

Living Questions

INTRODUCTION

Our interest in relationship and a relational ethic comes from the deep belief that we must not consider the person only as an object. As we treat the body, we treat the soul. As we treat the mechanical heart, we treat the feeling heart; as we treat the feeling heart, we also treat the mechanical heart. As Hans-George Gadamer wrote, the interconnection of body and soul vividly shows the "absolute inseparability of the living body and life itself."[1] This means that every action, every interaction, needs to attend to the ethical question of how we should treat each other. Especially when we understand that the word therapy is a derivative of the Greek *therapeia*, meaning "service,"[2] we see the importance of questioning our action, our treatment or therapy, from a moral view. As action has to do with relationship, we realize that relationship is key to ethical action. Relationship and its focus on the whole, "the whole of being,"[3] is so essential that it cannot be limited to the private world of individuals (the doctor-patient relationship), but is an ethic of service for all of humankind (individual-society-world). We have been asking throughout this text and, with Gadamer,[4] ask again, *What ought we to do? What ought science and its facilities for objectification mean to us? How can science, with its instrumentation of the human body, be connected once again to our lived experience? What needs*

*to change so that experience of one's own individuality is not
irrevocably lost in the context of modern data banks located
in the house that technology has built? How does the house of
technology define who we are and what we are capable of
achieving?* Questioning leads us on.

We know this house of technology. From the club or spear,
pot, wheel, printing press, birth control pill, and now the internet, we have reached a point where we cannot be educated
without a computer, cannot get around without a car, cannot
communicate without a telephone, fax, or e-mail. As Ursula
Franklin says, "The house is continually being extended and
remodelled. More and more of human life takes place within
its walls, so that today there is hardly any human activity that
does not occur within this house. All of us are affected by the
design of this house, by the division of its space, by the location of its doors and walls."[5] In the 1990 Massey Lectures,
Franklin, one of Canada's outstanding scientists, spoke about
her concerns regarding our technical house. We know that
the "healthcare room" in our house of technology is particularly remarkable, with its breathtaking advances in what technology can do for us. Newspapers flash headlines: "Stem Cells
Provide Hope," "Man Lives with an Artificial Heart," "A Sheep
is Cloned," "Human Gene is Planted into a Pig Heart for
Xenotransplantation," "People in Isolated Communities Get
Psychiatric Help through Interactive TV," and "Babies Born
Weighing as Little as 500 Grams Live." But technology can
also do other things: "A Badly Beaten Baby Is Kept on Life
Supports so that the Father Will Not Be Charged with Murder," "We Can Get Rid of Girls," and "Why Can't Human Organs Be Bought and Sold?" Franklin notes, "The values of
technology have so permeated the public mind that all too
frequently what is efficient is seen as the right thing to do."[6]
Bruce Phillips, Canada's Privacy Commissioner, warns, "if we
let technology become our god, we will certainly become
technology's sheep."[7]

We have come to live so naturally in the house that technology built (whether our homes, our hospitals, our schools,
our cities) that we hardly notice. It is so easy to think that
technology is a mere tool, a neutral device without any value
of its own. Such easy acceptance of this tool has put us into a

technological trance so that we hardly notice its moral impact. Although sometimes it is not easily found, we do believe there is an important room for ethics in the house of technology.

ROOM FOR ETHICS QUESTIONS

The job of ethics is to notice, to ask questions, to challenge the taken-for-granted, which might even break the trance. Is the house of technology where we want to live? Is this the kind of home we want for our children? The challenge of ethics is to ask questions about how to use technology and its instrumentation in what Robert Bruch calls a "properly human context."[8] How do we keep our house of technology in order? This house of technology, with its room for ethical contemplation, is our commons. It is found both in the familiar practices of the private house as well as in the world where people are at home together.[9] We have a house that has become so automated, bureaucratized, and technologized that there may be a need to reflect on how technology can be brought back into the service of what Gadamer called "that fundamental rhythm which sustains the proper order of bodily life."[10] The flow of the living body as it restores its rhythms—from loss of balance to new forms of stability, from illness to recovery, from life to death—needs our attention. This flow is the breath—the inspiration and expiration—that has been woven throughout our text: the breathing together, the catching our breath, the breathing body, breathing the same air, breathing in ethical tension, and breathing out ethical action. Breath, from Indo-European *bhreu*, means to bubble or boil, pointing to its derivatives of cooking or brewing.[11] Breath is life. Breath brings us back to the flow and rhythm of nature, the nature of home. What kind of house do we want to inhabit? How do we want to dwell? First, a story.

GATHERING AROUND THE HOUSE

Sue Bender relates this story. Once upon a time on a remote Japanese island, there lived a monk, Ekai.[12] At his monastery, there was no electricity, phone, or TV—and no car.

This monk, Ekai, had a beaming, open face with a shiny shaven head and clear, electric eyes. He spoke with great pleasure of the challenging tasks of training monks, supervising the building of a new temple, and his work with the surrounding community. The monks had a simple schedule. Several times a week they walked down the steep mountain to a small village where they waited for a bus that would take them into town. They bought supplies and fresh vegetables, just what they could carry on their backs, took the bus back to the village, and then walked back up the mountain. It was a balanced life of possibilities and limits. Then, a local supporter of the temple, hoping to make the monks' lives easier, gave the community a gift, a small minivan. Now, when Ekai is asked, "How are you and how are things going at the temple?" he says, "Wonderful and hard." "I feel the car is running me," he says. "Now I seem to go up and down the mountain too many times. There is even more to do—too much," he shrugs. "I love to work in the kitchen, but lately I've been too busy with all this work around the car. I can see that the kitchen isn't working." And then he sighs, and adds, "Life doesn't work when the kitchen doesn't work." The house that technology built, which offers us a car—and a CAT scan, a smart card, reproductive technology, laptops, the internet—is exciting and enhancing, even entrancing, efficient, expedient. In our story of Ekai, the car, the metaphor of technological life, is contrasted with the kitchen as metaphor of ethical human life. This example is simplistic, but can be instructive. How can we again feel "at home" in our world? How do we want to live?

Think again of intensive-care units where machines are central to the environment—about over-treatments that patients receive, treatments administered by professionals who may not want them for themselves. The technology is there to be used. It is hard to know when to stop. When technology takes over, there is danger that professionals become mere objects, managed and controlled, as means to accomplish technological ends.[13] Think of the smart card, that magical card, the size of a credit card that will hold medical history and family information to improve patient care, reduce administrative costs, and prevent duplication of services. The most obvious questions about smart cards are about confidentiality and privacy of information: *Who will have access to them?* (professionals, insurance companies, employment administrators, social services); *How will one protect access?* Think of going to the pharmacy to pick up an antibiotic for some kind of infection. You give the pharmacist your smart card, because you want to make sure that the drugs you are taking will not be incompatible. In filling out the prescription, the pharmacist says, "Oh, I see your doctor says you have a bit of eczema; would you like to pick up some cream for it as well?"[14]

Think of the very distraught man who comes into the emergency room with a badly broken finger. Not a problem, easily managed, easily treated—not a priority; this injury is way down on the list of illnesses such as heart disease or cancer. But with the knowledge that this man is a concert pianist, the broken finger takes on a dimension we did not understand initially. When we allow technology to direct human action and to separate knowledge and experience, separate the person from the body part, there is danger of cultivating "insensitivity, a clinical detachment, a deadening of emotions," and when we do that, says Samuel Blumenfeld, "we begin to lose our way, to be less human."[15]

In this chapter, we will explore the technological house of healthcare, to uncover current cracks in its structure, so that we can build a stronger foundation based on our relationships to each other. Using the example of the developing ethos of the medical profession—codes, valuing of objectification, professionalism, and the marketplace—we will show the need to heed the call of relationship precisely because ethics has meaning through relationship.[16] First we will explore the history of ethics that dates back to Hippocrates.

PROFESSIONAL CODES

For many older physicians, the ethical commitment of medicine was expressed in the doctor-patient relationship, although little attention was given to the nature of this relationship prior to the last half of the twentieth century. Medical ethics, as such, was not taught to medical students prior to this. Perhaps the closest to a course in ethics were lectures on forensic medicine and its legal context. The ethos of the profession lay in the respect for the prudence and erudition of one's preceptors in the "noble art"—a largely unexpressed but mutually understood ethos. The preceptors, for their part, were assumed to express these concepts (which were as much etiquette as ethics) through their behavior toward their patients and colleagues. In the last five decades, all of this has changed. Some of the factors influencing this change are increased knowledge of medical science, specialization and compartmentalization, diagnostic ability, public funding, a shift to hospital care, medical research, and distancing between individual patients and their personal physicians. The attitudes built into past medical education can be derived from the Hippocratic Oath (circa 500 BCE).[17]

We highlight some of the main precepts included in this oath. It begins,

I swear by Apollo Physician and Aesculapius . . . that I will fulfil according to my ability and judgement this oath and this covenant. I will:

- hold him who has taught me this art as equal to my parents and to live my life in partnership with him, and if he is in need of money to give him a share of mine, and to regard his offspring as equal to my brothers in male lineage.
- keep them [the sick] from harm and injustice.
- neither give a deadly drug to anybody if asked for it, nor will I make a suggestion to this effect. Similarly I will not give to a woman an abortive remedy.
- come for the benefit of the sick, remaining free of all intentional injustice, of all mischief and in particular of sexual relations with both female and male persons, be they free or slaves.
- what I may see or hear in the course of the treatment in regard to the life of men, which on no account one must spread abroad, I will keep to myself holding such things shameful to be spoken about.

If I fulfill this oath and do not violate it, may it be granted to me to enjoy life and art, being honored with fame among all men for all time to come; if I transgress it and swear falsely, may the opposite of all this be my lot.

There are many good points in this code, which include acting with beneficence towards the sick, doing no harm (*primum non nocere*), acting to preserve patients' privacy and to preserve disclosed information as confidential, and acting virtuously at all times. The ethically flawed points include paternalism, incomplete disclosure of medical facts concerning outcomes, a lack of concept of informed consent, and no concept of patients' autonomy or participatory decision making. While the historic Hippocratic Oath had no contemporary official sanction by the profession, it was accepted until recent decades as a cornerstone of physicians' behavior in framing the physician-patient relationship. Subsequent medical codes—such as those of Maimomides, Thomas Perceval, and the first code of the American Medical Association (1845)—purport to give a new perspective on the behavior of physicians, although this is not too evident in the following quotation from Perceval: "Physicians and surgeons should minister to the sick, reflecting that the ease, health, and lives of those committed to their charge depend on their skills, attention, and fidelity. . . . They should study, in their deportment, so to unite tenderness with steadiness, and condescension with authority, as to inspire the minds of their patients with gratitude, respect, and confidence."[18] Over the years a pervasive "heroic" hierarchy[19] developed, in which the doctor remained active, knowledgeable, and authoritative, and the patient and family were seen as passive, ignorant, and dependent. This Aesculapian authority was based on the knowledge and expertise of doctors, to which patients and families were expected to comply by taking the subordinate "sick role." These interlocking notions are explicit in the Hippocratic Oath, and may still be implicit in the ethics of some contemporary medical associations. As one of the doctors, a member of our research group said during our research: *The code was taught in medical school by seniors who learned it from their seniors who learned it from their seniors. Doctors were trained to be of use to people and reach*

beyond emotions and feelings—to not let emotions stand
in the way of helping people. Emotions were expressed at
home—anger, fear, great sadness—but at work, doctors
have to be of use![20]

The belief that doctors and other experts must maintain authority is found in the distancing that was first articulated in
codes with the pushing off of emotions and feelings.

Consider some of the precepts in the 1996 iteration of the
Code of Ethics of the Canadian Medical Association, as illustrated by 12 of its 43 ethical statements.[21] This version of the
code is also noteworthy, in that it was the first time that the
code was stated in gender-neutral language—all previous edi-
tions assumed that physicians were male.

- Treat all patients with respect; do not exploit them for
  personal advantage.
- Do not discriminate against any patient on such
  grounds as age, gender, marital status, medical condition, national or ethnic origin, physical or mental disability, . . . sexual orientation, or socio-economic status.
- Make every reasonable effort to communicate with your
  patients in such a way that information exchanged is
  understood.
- Respect the right of the competent patient to accept or
  reject any medical care recommended.
- Respect the intentions of an incompetent patient as
  they were expressed (e.g., through an advance directive or proxy designation) before the patient became
  incompetent.
- Inform the potential research subject, or proxy, about
  the purpose of a (research) study, its source of funding, the nature of possible harms and benefits, and the
  nature of your participation.
- Refuse to participate in or support practices that violate basic human rights.
- Collaborate with other physicians and health professionals in the care of patients and the functioning and
  improvement of health services.

This contemporary code of medical ethics reflects a move to a partnership with patients. But perhaps one can only expect a code to represent a summary of the *principles* of ethics because they reflect behavior in a universal way. In practice, codes are actualized in our demeanor and so they are found useful in professional life. Yet, in spite of the importance and values embedded in professional codes of ethics, *codes, by themselves, are not enough to ensure ethical practice.*

OBJECTIVE KNOWLEDGE
AND PROFESSIONALISM

The development of medical knowledge credits the scientific method and the value that is placed on objective knowledge.[22] Maintaining objectivity is important because different professionals come from various experiential, religious, ethical, and moral backgrounds, which in turn influence practice situations. It is not unusual for professionals to disagree on how to approach different situations, so that maintaining objectivity and professional distance is valued and is felt to be appropriate. Theoretical scientific knowledge is thought to be universal, and timeless, and therefore True, with a capital "T."[23] Objective knowledge strives for generalizability and predictability, which lead to control of life and prevent unhappy surprises. Objective knowledge strives to keep ambiguity and uncertainty away. Such knowledge is very tempting to both develop and to use, as it gives a sense of security that life can, in fact, be controlled. With this objective knowledge, we are able most easily to carry our professional practice, doing what we have been taught, and fulfilling our social obligations to provide the best care possible. In standing back in objective distance, we hold emotions at bay so that they do not interfere with our ability to make clear and rational decisions.

Professionalism and distance are credited with helping to define who professionals are, what work they ought to do, what their rightful place in society ought to be, and how they may best respond in uniform ways to particular cues. Because the work that professionals do is demanding, procedures, theories, and technologies facilitate greater efficiency and effectiveness. The demands of procedures and duties of professional practice are made easier by holding at a distance, so that ethical issues are resolved simply by following the rules. Much of the teaching we receive as doctors, nurses, and other professionals occurs without our being taught the theoretical foundations, terminology, and philosophy that underpins the teaching. Rather, there is teaching by mentors within practice; for example, watching doctors interact with patients. Students recognize that they learn ethical knowledge by being in the room, listening to the dialogue between the patient, the family, the doctor, and the nurse. Often such experiences make profound and lasting impressions. Here is one example that jolted a physician in our research group to think more about ethics:

> I remember when I was an intern, one of the first nights that I was on call, we got called for a cardiac arrest on an 85-year-old woman with terminal cancer. And we all pounded on her chest and took turns et cetera. Suddenly I said to myself, what are we doing? Well, we've got technology. We've got techniques. We do it. We've really embraced that.[24]

Ethical questions are experienced in day-to-day life.

Just as we have a desire for knowledge that is factual and certain for *clinical* use, so we also have a desire for the certainty of knowledge for *ethical* use. This desire has led to the formation of a cadre of professional ethicists whose job it is to dispense knowledge that enables us to move to ethical certainty. This seems to be the goal of "applied ethics." Principle-driven ethics are part of this approach to develop ethical knowledge that can be applied as clinical knowledge has been. Sometimes theoretical approaches, such as those based on abstract concepts such as autonomy, beneficence, non-maleficence, and justice, when they are divorced from clinical practice, may create distance between caregivers and their patients or clients. Of course, ethical principles are attractive within the ethos of professionalism, because they purport to resolve issues by following a set of "rules" that tend to place professionals in a controlling position.[25]

THE MARKETPLACE

During the first years of our research, the Canadian health-care system was downsized, leaving many professionals wondering about their own jobs, as well as wondering about how they were going to look after patients. Many caregivers felt they were "run off their feet," and, as a result, felt demoralized and undervalued. It seemed that the "bottom line" of efficiency and expediency was emphasized without proper attention to how people were affected. Currently, commercialization and corporatization represent an increasingly dominant economic paradigm that is turning medicine and healthcare into a medical-industrial complex.[26] Normative values of compassion and care may be lost when profit becomes the end of medicine. "The medical profession seems to have lost its soul," says the physician Solomon Benatar, "with greed being turned into a virtue under the influence of powerful medical corporations."[27] Accumulation of wealth through the exploitation of human vulnerability in illness may become an "end in itself" for healthcare services. With this focus on economics, there is danger that we, as a people, may lose our commitment and connection to each other, and even our connection to the earth. Emphasis on the marketplace can result in sloth (a moral torpor where we pass by on the other side) and greed (when some have salaries beyond anything one can consume and use), which, as John MacLuchlan Gray says, has led to the sorrow and violence experienced throughout the world.[28] The totalizing of all forms of life into economics that serves the desires of multinational corporations and stockholders leads to inequities of wealth, construction of violence through the logic of self-interest, and the destruction of freedom and democratic participation of all in the construction of shared futures.[29]

When the ethos of medicine is replaced by an ethos of business, individual patients as well as whole populations are adversely affected. In a healthcare system dominated by the powerful ideology of the marketplace, both doctors and patients become commodified—both are dominated by the procedural and business priorities of corporate managers. Not only are we dealing with the human suffering related to disease, injury, suffering, and death, we are caught in the desire to make perfect everything about ourselves and our lives—cosmetic surgery, genetic enhancement for athletic advantage, and so on. The biomedical model related to disability, as discussed in chapter six, with its emphasis on prevention, places individuals without those potentials in a position of vulnerability, discrimination, and oppression.

While professional codes, the objectivity of knowledge, and the careful and efficient use of limited resources are ethically important, we, in this text, call us back to a thoughtful consideration of the whole person and attention to the connections between whole persons. The more that our health-care system slips into depersonalization, the more inept our care will become. We sometimes think that sticking to the limits of objective knowledge is easier and quicker, but we have found that, in the long run, it is not. There is too great a potential for our care to become demeaning or to be wrong. While we all have been in situations in which we want an expert to tell us what to do, more often we experience experts as persons who do not pay attention to seeing or hearing us as we understand ourselves to be. The call to meaningful human relationship is the task of ethics. As David Geoffrey Smith says, "Life calls us, draws us into its fullness, its complexities, as the means through which we find ourselves to be human." [30] Life calls us to be human, to be of the earth, to be in relation to the earth and each other.

THE CALL TO RELATIONSHIP

The challenge of ethics is to keep alive the question of human values in our house that technology has built, to keep attention on any cracks in the walls of our house that we might not otherwise notice. Like the monk Ekai, we want to make sure that the kitchen is still working. Kitchens, centers of nourishment (where we can talk with family and friends, learn to share, laugh and cry, and just to be) are transformative places, where separate ingredients are mixed together, put into the oven, and something entirely different, something new. In the transformation to something new, one can no longer identify the separate ingredients, such as flour, salt, or eggs. Of course kitchens are filled with modern tools, but when we think of a kitchen we often think of it as a place of warmth, sharing, and conversation, fostering growth and fulfilling commitments. Here, attention to the kitchen means attending to human experience—the place where we dwell. Here we recover our moral language. Here we attend to relationships. It is often around the kitchen table that we learn who we are and who we want to be. It is life that calls us.

How can we foster ethical and moral relationships? It might be as simple as taking our attention away from the computer screen to enter into conversation with the patient who is connected to that screen. Of course, we know that maintaining relations in healthcare is difficult (and may even become impossible) when resources are limited so that there are not enough doctors, nurses, or other staff; there is not enough time; and when the notion of strangers treating strangers is taken as a given, rather than an idea to be resisted. When we focus on relationships, we recognize how our technical house can restrict reciprocity and reduce healthy human contact. We need to build ways to foster dialogue between professionals and patients, among professionals themselves, and among all of us who live in this community—to know each other—to decide on our common human ends.

While this text hopes to promote a calling back to relationship, we recognize that relationship is not something that can be mandated. A "call" is not a mandate. *To call* means to cry out in a loud voice, to summon, to awaken, to name, to bring to action.[31] In this text, we have persistently called attention to relationship as an ethical responsibility. One way to respond to the call of relationship is to broaden the conversation of ethics—to get us all involved in discussion about issues in our healthcare and medical world. But conversation needs language, and we need to recover a language that can open the notion of being at home in our world—home not only in the car, but also in the kitchen. Rather then leaving it to a panel of experts to proclaim the Truth with a capital "T," our call is to attend to relationship in all its complexities.

One way is to let go of any preconceived "script" to more fully engage one another.

LETTING GO OF THE SCRIPT

In 1998, we put together a presentation for the Canadian Bioethics Society to explore the relationship between principle-based and relational ethics. The original idea was to have one person give the case, another to give 20 minutes of ethical principles, another to give 20 minutes on relationship, and another to give 20 minutes leading the discussion. That would be the workshop. We found, however, that the only way to present relational ethics is in an interactive way, with us talking together with the audience—which would screw up the script. Perhaps, we thought, with a relational approach to ethics we *do* have to let go of the script. "Letting go of the script" of health ethics or bioethics is challenging, and requires self-reflection, negotiation, risk-taking, and change. Letting go, however, is not about abandoning what we already know, such as ethical theory or principles. Rather, letting go is about shaking our selves free of the beliefs, practices, and traditions that restrain our ideas. In letting go, we open ourselves to broadening our commitments to rationality, which includes emotions and intuitions. In letting go of the script, we search for the questions as much as the answers.[32] We become involved in the act of discovery.

In drama, the script gives careful direction to the setting, the lines, and tone of voice, within a carefully crafted narrative. The drama, if well-written, leads to specific outcomes that both actors and those in the audience find satisfying. We think of the script as an authority, so it may not really matter who the actors are. People in the audience, as observers, are comfortable that the right words will be said at the right time. But the drama only comes to life when the actors let the script go, to the extent that they *become* the characters. When the actors inhabit and *live* the words they say, then both audience and actors are drawn into drama. For actors, it might take time to be comfortable with the scripted lines—for the words to become "my" words, the action, "my" action, and the story, "my" story. To let go of the script does not mean "screwing up"—like forgetting a line or making some other mistake. To let go involves being present in the moment, being present in the role, and being present to the other actors. In letting go of the script, we become like jazz musicians whose careful attention and response to each other creates the resulting complex music. Such music comes from respectful attention, knowledge, and trust in each other, as other musicians. Even in a symphony, a musical score serves as the bare bones or the principles to be fleshed out by interpreting the composer's intention in a unique and original way. When one lets go of the script, the outcomes may not be completely known ahead of time.

Each summer in Edmonton, *The Fringe Festival* opens its playhouses and streets for a 10-day period for innovative drama. Plays and performances of all types are held in various venues in the heart of the city. The excitement and festival feelings are heightened by street performers, food venues, and long lines of people waiting for one play to end and the next to begin. Many of the plays are carefully scripted, and the success of the plays has to do in part with how well the actors inhabit their roles. One interactive drama attempts to increase awareness about the lives of street kids. *Katie is Missing* is both the title and the problem.[33] It is up to the Fringe Festival audience to help find her. In doing so they, themselves, become actors in the drama. These audience-actors can decide where to go to find Katie. Should they look for her through her alcoholic and abusive mother? Should they search for her drug dealer or her couch-potato stepfather? Should they go to the police? Having prepared a number of script possibilities, the actors on the stage follow the guidance of the actors in the audience. Stephen Liley, a young playwright and youth worker, wrote and produced this play that was performed in the street—the home of the characters. Like the characters in the play, the actors are from a Youth Co-op that provides a safe place and counseling for homeless youth. These young actors have little stage experience but come with a full experience of life on the street. The play invites community people to get involved in the issues and dilemmas of youth.

"People usually don't even notice these kids," says Liley, "They just walk on by."[34] But here not only does the paying audience get involved, but so do people walking on the street. One night, during a tense moment when the actors shouted to each other about the missing Katie, a passer-by with a cell phone called out, "Should I call the police?"—a Good Samaritan with a cell phone.

But letting go of the script is not easy. Relationship is not easy. Relationship is not about holding another's hand, having a good bedside manner, or even being willing to use one's cell phone. The complexities of relationship are real, and we wonder, at times, if it evokes an ideal that cannot be accomplished. Perhaps relational ethics can only be a call—a call to pay increased attention to how we are with each other—to imagine how to make life whole. Perhaps relational ethics is the way we live ethical questions. Can we imagine what the genetic revolution may do to our relationships? If a child is born with five parents' names on the birth certificate (sperm donor, egg donor, surrogate mother, adoptive mother, and adoptive father) could we imagine ways that love is still at the center of the care for the child? If we cannot, what ethic will govern these relationships? Can we imagine how technologies can support relations? Can we imagine attention to relations as our first ethical concern? These are important questions, and it is time to grapple with the ethical complexities that surround us.

In the call to relationship, within the medical and healthcare environment and in other spheres of life, we have considered a number of themes. In many ways the call to relationship is a reminder of what we already know and do. Because relationship is never a past accomplishment, but always under construction, the call is seen as an invitation to return to relationship—or dare we say love—as our supreme ethic. In our research, we developed themes that point to the kind of relations we see as important between doctors and patients, nurses and patients, in all healthcare relationships. It is in the space of relationship, whether it is within the caregiver and patient relationship or between individuals and agencies and the like, where we find the themes of the relational ethic: engagement, mutual respect, embodiment, and environment. Can these themes help us consider how to live a relational ethic in the house of technology?

ENGAGEMENT:
CLOSE-UP OR DISTANT

Raymond Duff succinctly outlined the difference between concepts of "distant ethics" and "close-up ethics."[35] We believe that Duff's close-up ethics resonates with our work in relational ethics. Duff begins with the clear statement that "people are social beings by design, not by choice," to remind us that we are born into relationship.[36] The choice is not whether we will be engaged, but is how we are to enact those relationships. According to Duff, close-up ethics directs attention to the specific family, religious, philosophical, or social conditions or orientations that commonly serve as the foundation for individual and family life. It draws attention to the whole person, and requires active participation between professionals, patients, and families in deciding for and providing care. As such, it moves away from the prescribed codes of organized religious, philosophical, legal, or even health ethics directives. Rather, as Duff says, "it rightly gives people, both as individual and social beings a major voice in shaping their own lives. And it holds them responsible for the consequences."[37] Close-up or relational ethics is difficult to practice, because it is founded on empathy and education, rather than on knowledge and principles. While its practice is demanding, it gives power to both patients and families, on the one hand, and health professionals on the other, as people who exercise responsibility, and, in that exercise, tend to become stronger. The reciprocal nature of relational ethics speaks to the conversation that must occur between people.

In contrast to this more close-up approach to ethics, Duff says that "distant ethics" gives emphasis to abstract ethical principles, stereotypes, and rules derived from religious, philosophical, scientific, and legal analyses. Distant ethics, in Duff's terms, brings foreign or alien forms of reasoning into the lives of people, reasoning that may be opposed to the personal beliefs and conscience of individuals, their families, and particular religious or health advisors. This conflict in forms of reasoning may silence patients and families and make it easier for them to take a passive role. Practitioners, who may often try to practice a relational ethic, are often inclined, indeed, are often encouraged to practice a more formal distant ethics, as Duff says, "because of a modern pre-occupation with rights and individualism . . . [that] disallows systematic acknowledgment of the habits of the heart, of people as social beings."[38] Distant ethics excludes attention to many relevant facts, such as how patients, families, and other health professionals feel about the problems they face. Distant ethics concentrates on professional knowledge and reasoning, which do not acknowledge the limits and weaknesses of professions. Often in distant ethics there is little or no recognition of the strengths and abilities of patients or clients.

Duff, in referring to the work of Ronald Preston, points out that both the modern doctor and the modern public place an extremely high value on "aspirational heroism," which seeks, through application of science and technology, to control, if not defeat, disease and death. This orientation provides a magnificent sense of power for health professionals and the institutions through which they work. It is true that we, as a society, may lap up the magic pill of aspirational heroism, but Eric Cassell believes that "humble heroism," a more close-up approach to ethics, consists of steadfastness, duty, and loyalty, which are all necessary for dealing with adversity and suffering.[39] Like Duff, the relational ethics project supports attention to close-up ethics as the best approach to expressing the relationship between those involved in healthcare.

MUTUAL RESPECT:
SOCIAL OR PERSONAL

The healthcare relation, in the context of close-up ethics, acknowledges that both professionals and patients give of themselves. Patients disclose their feelings of vulnerability, discomfort, anxiety, and pain. Caregivers accept disclosures by patients and treat all aspects of it with respect. In return, patients reciprocate by respecting the openness and willingness of professionals to "be with them" in their vulnerability. This mutual respect enriches the relationship in ways that are not evident in more formal, distant relationships, which can be accentuated by the formality of the "white coat," the "desk in between," the "stethoscope neck-tie." Even the current practice of patients going to the hospital or clinic (the home of the professional) is a radical change from when the professional visited as a guest in patients' homes. Now, patients wait (often for long periods) upon the favor of the professional at the hospital or clinic. More recent moves to home care (a long tradition in public health nursing) have been influenced by the need for close-up and personal relations of professionals and patients, more easily experienced in the home. In order, though, for home care to be able to foster relations, resources (both financial and personal) need greater attention.

Some insights in considering the call to relationship come from John Macmurray's analysis of types of relationship.[40] Macmurray makes a clear distinction between social relationships and personal relationships. In social relationships, "we suppress, for the time being at least, the fullness and wholeness of our natures,"[41] and associate with the other for a specific purpose or function that has an achievable given end— such as with a car mechanic or a real estate agent. "Out of this there springs a life of social co-operation through which we can provide for our common needs, and achieve common ends," Macmurray notes.[42] The functional nature of social relationships means that we cannot enter into this form of relationship with our whole selves, as complex persons, because the purpose involved is only, in general, one of our life purposes. In contrast to this notion of social relationship, Macmurray discusses personal relationships. In personal relations, we express our whole selves to one another in mutuality and fellowship. "It is difficult to find a word to express this kind of relationship which will convey its full meaning," Macmurray says, "not because there are no words, but because they have all been specialized and degraded by misuse.

Friendship, fellowship, communion, love, are all in one way
or another liable to convey a false or partial meaning."[43]

A society is made up of persons in social relationships
who have a particular function. Personal relationships are between persons *as* persons. They may have little to do with
any coincident-shared function. As Macmurray puts it, "A
personal relation is a relation of equality, and it exists for the
realization and expression of *freedom*"—not only as a social
function.[44] "Morality depends, in this relationship as in all
others, on our ability to treat one another always as persons,
and the differences between us as the means for realizing and
expressing and enjoying our common personality."[45]

If we accept these two broad categorizations of relationship, what, we should ask, is the nature of the professional
relationship between health professionals and the people cared
for? Already, in such an analysis as this, we can become dis-
satisfied with the phrase "doctor-patient," because it can have
the connotation of distant ethics. Would we find the words
"doctor with the patient" better? Not really, as neither "doctor" nor "patient" is present in all healthcare relations. There
are many health professionals, each with important and unique
abilities and skills. Further, not all persons who access health
services are adequately described by the word "patient." In
fact, the use of words like client, consumer, and customer are
prominent in healthcare, and suggest a different kind of relation than the word "patient." Professional relationships in
healthcare are complex and differ in ways described in this
chapter—as well as in this book, in general—from relationships between persons in most of the nonhealthcare professions—most of which are social relationships (in the sense
that Macmurray uses this decription): "All persons are equal;
and this is the first law of the personal life. It does not mean
that there are not immense differences between one person
and another: it means that these differences have no bearing
upon the possibility of personal relations."[46]

In this discussion, we refer to the broad categories of relationship with professionals and patients and professionals
with each other. In the healthcare relationship, persons share
their physical and emotional needs, which involve sharing

thoughts, aspirations, frustrations, and limitations. By such sharing, the personal relationship is recognized. All persons need to be treated as moral equals and enjoy the freedom of a personal relationship with professionals in ways that clients in other types of (nonhealthcare) professional relationships do not expect or need. In the healthcare relationship, all must respect the vulnerability of the other and respect the necessity of personal relationship. In healthcare situations, caregivers and patients enter the encounter from a place of "prejudgment" or "foreknowledge" from which to encounter the other.[47] It is with this prior knowledge (healthcare knowledge, expertise, experience, values, and beliefs) that we can begin the process of coming to a shared understanding—to produce an understanding that might be new for both.

EMBODIMENT:
THINKING OR FEELING

Healthcare is a place where knowledge is "full-blooded." In this place, it is not just facts (biological, religious, or social) that need attention, but the deeply significant facets of lived lives, as people respond to the effects of health and illness. In a very real way, relational knowledge is embodied—it is *who we are* as much as what we do that is important. We embody our commitments—as father, mother, neighbor, doctor, or nurse. Because embodiment is such a difficult concept to understand, we again use a story. This is a story that Olive Schreiner told in 1890 about an artist.[48] While other artists painted with colors that were richer and rarer and painted more notable pictures, this artist, our artist, had only painted with one color—a color with a wonderful red glow. To find the secret, other artists sought costly and rare pigments from far away places or searched old books, but the red in their paintings faded after time. Our artist painted on and on, and as his hair grew whiter and whiter, his painting became redder and redder. One day our painter was found dead before his painting. When he was undressed, a mark of a wound was found above his left breast. After he was buried, people still wondered about where his color came from, and although the

artist was forgotten, his work lived on. Like the artist, whole
persons give of themselves to others, not from the dispassionate logic of reason, but from the embodied reason of passion.
Passion, here, is not the experience of runaway emotion, nor
the physical pleading in the name of passion, but of living life
in a full-bodied way.

Within the knowledge of embodiment, there is great need
for healthcare caregivers to attend to their own health and
well-being. We need to be watchful that giving in a full-bodied way does not lead to depletion and "burnout" of personal
energy, spirit, and happiness. We, as healthcare providers, need
to take care of ourselves as we care for others. We have discussed throughout the book that reciprocal relationships and
mutual respect demand care and respect for ourselves as we
care and respect others. Careful attention to our embodied
experience, that is, self-knowledge, tells us when we need to
talk to a colleague, have a coffee break, take a vacation, or do
other activities of self-renewal.

The nature of the healthcare relation is that it has less pre-
dictable outcomes than other relations—the unexpected reaction, the unusual complication, the tragic nature of some of
the experiences. There is almost always emotional tension in
such relationships—no matter how much experience the professional has, or how much the person tries to buffet the gusts
and storms of personal adversity. This tension is always there.
Thus, these healthcare relationships must always have these
uncertainties as part of their lived experience.

ENVIRONMENT: HERE AND THERE

The public at large and those in the health professions all
share an interest in the healthcare environment. In those countries where healthcare is publicly funded, every citizen is
aware that it is valuable, that it is available equally to all, and
that it is costly. It is also acknowledged that there are rising
costs in the areas of new technologies, new pharmaceuticals,
and ever-increasing public expectations. This is not the place
to enter into the healthcare debate, even though public polls
in Canada report that the issue is the top priority of Canadi-
ans as a whole. But there is common ground between the prin-

ciples of the public healthcare system and the practice of relational ethics by health professionals.

Healthcare, as we see it, is not a commodity, but a vital component of how, in Canada at least, the majority of citizens wish to look upon their fellow beings, in a rare expression of common concern, each for the other. This is a natural extension of relation at the individual level—the healthcare relation. Individual freedom must not be set against the common good, as individual freedom *is* the common good. We cannot believe that what is important "here" is different than what is important "there." We are in this together. As Jackie Hanagan wrote, "My welfare is tied up with the welfare of everyone in my society, my health is everyone's health. We share the water, the air, and the land."[49] We breathe the same air. We therefore feel strongly committed to preserving this shared healthcare environment. We dwell in the present—the shared world. Within this global concept, David Geoffrey Smith identifies the need for three kinds of truth: personal truth, truth as shared, and finding truth as finding home.[50] "If there is to be truth in the world, it will be only truth as shared, something between us. Such is the foundation of ethics in the age of globalization."[51] More complex is Smith's notion of truth as *home*, where "the practice of truth is nothing less than the practice of finding oneself at home in the world."[52]

FINDING THE WORLD AS HOME

As Hans-George Gadamer writes, the challenge of finding our home in the world, of being at home in the world, "includes not only the ability to manage by one's self, but also the ability to manage along with other people [which is] . . . a collective responsibility and in a genuinely shared existence both with and for one another."[53] Again, we ask with Gadamer, how our house of technology, with all its autonomated, bureaucratized, and mechanical apparatus, can be brought back into the service of our household, the place where we properly learn to integrate reliance and consideration for one another into our own lived existence.[54] "The house is what is held in common, it is both the familiar practices and the dwelling place where people are at home together."[55] The kind of good housekeeping that Gadamer talks about is the need to raise the sense of responsibility that goes beyond ourselves to take place across the planet as a whole: "The challenge is a continual one of sustaining our own internal balance within a larger social whole which requires both cooperation and participation ... to discover new possibilities for a more humane arrangement of things as they have been developed in our instrumentalized social organization."[56] This we can only do in conversation with others.

KEEPING THE
CONVERSATION GOING

The call to relationship is a call to dialogue. Early on in our research, we decided that one of many outcomes of this work is to keep the conversation going. Listening, hearing, giving, and receiving is ongoing. With an ethic of relationship, our task is to search for understanding, to find the middle ground, and to avoid entrenchment into ideology. Only then can we create space for new results—results opened by the imagination to foster growth and reduce suffering. There is no map or script in relational ethics to fall back on. We want to be sure that the advance directive or the smart card will encourage discussion and shared decision making, and not erode it (further); that they and other innovations will not disenfranchise people—neither the poor nor the rich, neither patients nor professionals. We propose that we attend to experience, share experience, and make time for authentic conversation about how we want to use technology in a properly human perspective. We do not want to cast away individual values and rights that have been built up over centuries of human experience—values that are fundamental to personal and social life. Rather, we want to place rights and values directly into a notion of relationship—the context of all life, responsibility for both self and other. Ethics reminds us to be attentive to both the car and to the kitchen in our house that technology has built. We want to consider what we can do to give renewed attention to the development of deep respect for each other, to foster tolerance and compassion, based on recognition that we all live in this house together. We need to choose, says Bruce Phillips, whether we will preserve our fundamental commitments to respect individuals as unique human beings (and to create viable, vibrant communities living in harmony), or whether we are prepared to offer ourselves up on the altar of technological domination.[57] Technology has built our modern house and we have the freedom to choose how we want to live in it.

This freedom is bound by our common life and the love we have for one another. As we act on our freedom, we need to keep living our questions of ethics: *How we should treat each other?* and *What are you going through?*

CONCLUSION

The research in relational ethics is ongoing, and reflects consistency with any project that asks questions about life as lived—ethics as lived. As David Geoffrey Smith says, coming to an understanding about how to live ethically in our changing world is "never a once-and-for-all event, but a continual process of emerging understanding, growing out of a spiralling dialectic between the parts and the whole."[58] From the situated center of the Relational Ethics Research Project, we identified four major themes, engagement, mutual respect, embodiment, and environment, that we used to discuss the nature of the ethical relation in healthcare. Attention to the relation-space offered us an opportunity to consider the importance of this space for ethical action, not only at the bedside, but within the world surrounding individual relations of two or more persons. We attempted to hear myriad voices through our attention to particular examples. That attention to difference and partiality recognizes the reality that no one voice can represent others; varied voices need to be heard and need to be interrupted and contradicted. This text has been one of emerging understanding of the need to respect relational space as an ethical responsibility, and therefore requires ongoing conversation with you, the reader, and with further research in the area. We invite continual conversation and continual attention to ethical relations in our healthcare world and in the larger world as our home. In fact, inviting and enacting continual conversation is our most important task.

NOTES

1. Hans-George Gadamer, *The Enigma of Health: The Art of Healing in a Scientific Age*, trans. Jason Gaiger and Nicholas Walker (Stanford, Calif.: Stanford University Press, 1996), 71.

2. Ibid., 128.

3. Ibid., 73.

4. Ibid., 71-72.

5. Ursula Franklin, *The Real World of Technology* (Concord, Ont.: Anansi, 1990), 11.

6. Ibid., 123.

7. Bruce Phillips, "Privacy or Service—Must We Be Forced to Choose?" (presentation to the New Brunswick Legislative Library Noon Hour Talk, Fredericton, N.B., 22 February 1996), 10.

8. Robert Burch, "Technology and Curriculum: Toward a Philosophical Perspective," (occasional paper no. 27, Department of Secondary Education, University of Alberta, Edmonton, Alb., 1984), 14.

9. See note 1 above, p. 79.

10. Ibid.

11. William Morris, ed., *The American Heritage Dictionary of the Ethics Language* (Boston: Houghton Mifflin, 1978), 1510.

12. Sue Bender, *Everyday Sacred: A Woman's Journey Home* (New York: HarperCollins, 1995), 30-33.

13. Sally Gadow, "Whose Body? Whose Story? The Question about Narrative in Women's Health Care," *Soundings* 77, no. 3-4 (1994): 295-307.

14. Sheri Alpert, "Smart Cards, Smarter Policy: Medical Records, Privacy, and Health Care Reform," *Hastings Center Report* 23, no. 6 (1993): 13-23, 17.

15. Samuel L. Blumenfeld, *The Retreat from Motherhood* (Boston: Beacon, 1975), 195.

16. Raymond Duff, " 'Close-up' versus 'Distant' Ethics: Deciding the Care of Infants with Poor Prognosis," *Seminars in Perinatology* 11, no. 3 (1987): 244-53, 244.

17. Jason Frasco, "Ancient Greek Medicine," 5 May 2002, *http://members.tripod.com/JFrazz9/med.html.*

18. Perceval, cited in Albert R. Jonsen, *The New Medicine*

and the Old Ethics (Cambridge, Mass.: Harvard University Press, 1990), 66. This statement was included in the American Medical Association *Code of Ethics* from 1847 to 1912.

19. See note 16 above.

20. Interdisciplinary Research Group #4.

21. Canadian Medical Association, *Code of Ethics of the Canadian Medical Association*, Ottawa, Ont., 15 October 1996, *http://www.cma.ca/inside/policybase/1996/10-15.htm.*

22. Ross Van Amburg, "A Copernican Revolution in Clinical Ethics: Engagement Versus Disengagement," *American Journal of Occupational Therapy* 51, no. 3 (1997): 186-90.

23. Lorraine Code, *What Can She Know? Feminist Theory and the Construction of Knowledge* (Ithaca, N.Y.: Cornell University Press, 1991), 242.

24. See note 20 above.

25. See note 17 above.

26. Solomon R. Benatar, "Just Healthcare Beyond Individualism: Challenges for North American Bioethics," *Cambridge Quarterly of Healthcare Ethics* 6, no. 4 (1997): 395-415.

27. Ibid., 407.

28. John MacLachlan Gray, "Beyond Good and Evil," (Toronto) *Globe and Mail*, 19 September 2001, R1, R4.

29. David Geoffrey Smith, "The Mission of the Hermeneutic Scholar," in *The Mission of the Hermeneutic Scholars: Essays in Honor of Nelson Haggerson*, ed. M. Wolfe (New York: Peter Lang, 2002), 183-99.

30. Ibid., 184.

31. See note 11 above, p. 190.

32. The authors acknowledge the contribution of Susan James and Hari China, members of the research group, for earlier drafts of the idea included in this section.

33. Darren Stewart, "A Dramatic Lesson in the Life of the Street," *Edmonton Journal*, 25 August 2001, B1, B8.

34. Ibid., B8.

35. See note 16 above.

36. Ibid., 244.

37. Ibid.

38. Ibid., 245.

39. Eric J. Cassell, "The Nature of Suffering and the Goals of Medicine," *New England Journal of Medicine* 306, no. 11 (1982): 639-45.

40. John Macmurray, *Reason and Emotion* (London, U.K.: Faber & Faber, 1935/1995).
	41. Ibid., 55.
	42. Ibid., 56.
	43. Ibid., 56.
	44. Ibid., 64.
	45. Ibid., 66.
	46. Ibid., 60.
	47. See note 29 above.
	48. Olive Schreiner, *Dreams* (London, U.K.: Unwin, 1890), 101-3.
	49. Jackie Flanagan, "Editorial," *Alberta Views*, 5, no. 3, (2002): 6.
	50. David Geoffrey Smith, *Teaching in Global Times* (Edmonton, Alb.: Pedagon Press, 2002), 34.
	51. Ibid., 38.
	52. Ibid., 39.
	53. See note 1 above, pp. 79, 82.
	54. Ibid.
	55. Ibid., 80.
	56. Ibid., 1.
	57. See note 7 above.
	58. See note 29 above, p. 186.

Appendix A

Interdisciplinary Research Group Members

PRINCIPAL INVESTIGATOR

Vangie Bergum, PhD, is a Professor in the John Dossetor Health Ethics Centre and the Faculty of Nursing, University of Alberta. Her background in childbirth education and public health nursing brought her to ethical questions in healthcare. She has published in both ethics and mothering from her research approach of hermeneutic phenomenology. Professor Bergum completed her term as director of the John Dossetor Health Ethics Centre in 2002.

CO-INVESTIGATOR

John Dossetor, MD, PhD, is Professor Emeritus with the University of Alberta. Prior to founding the Joint Faculties Bioethics Project at the University of Alberta in 1986, Dr. Dossetor had a long and successful career as a nephrologist and research scientist. His experiences in the early days of kidney transplantation raised his ethical awareness and eventually resulted in further study in ethics. Dr. Dossetor's work in medicine and bioethics was recognized in 1995 when he was appointed as an Officer of the Order of Canada. He currently lives in Ottawa, Ontario, where he continues to consult nationally and internationally on transplantation and ethics.

PROJECT COORDINATOR

Sandra MacPhail, MN, began work on the research project as a graduate student in 1993. Since that time she has completed a Masters in Nursing, with a thesis focus on ethics and community nursing. Besides coordinating this interdisciplinary study, she directs another multiphased qualitative study looking at women caregivers' support and nonsupport.

TEAM MEMBERS

Wendy Austin, RN, PhD, is a Professor in the Faculty of Nursing and the John Dossetor Health Ethics Centre, University of Alberta. She was involved in Phase I of the study and led the Mental Health subgroup in Phase II. She went on to investigate Mental Health Practitioners' Experience of Moral Distress in a study funded by the Social Sciences and Humanities Council (SSHRC) of Canada. She currently holds a Canada Research Chair in Relational Ethics in Healthcare.

John Stephen Bamforth, MD, is an Associate Professor in the Department of Medical Genetics, University of Alberta, and is past Director of the Medical Genetics Clinic at the University of Alberta Hospital. His interest in ethics has evolved from his genetics counseling practice. Dr. Bamforth led the Genetics subgroup in Phase II of the study.

Charles Bidwell, PhD, is an Ordained Minister and Educator. He is an expert in the use of instructional media and until his retirement was the Director of the Health Sciences Media Services and Development Department at the University of Alberta. He worked closely with the Faculty of Medicine in this capacity as Faculty Service Officer. Dr. Bidwell is now active as a consultant and is pursuing an interest in the dramatic arts.

Marion Briggs, BScPT, is a Physical Therapist who worked at the University of Alberta Hospitals and taught in the Faculties of Rehabilitation Medicine, Nursing, and Medicine, University of Alberta. She provided administrative leadership for a major redesign of patient care at the University of Alberta

Hospitals. She is the Coordinator of Program Planning and Development for the Department of Internal Medicine at the Eastern Virginia Medical School. She and Dr. Susan James collaborated in Phase II of the research in a subgroup looking at the ethical relationships between and among healthcare providers.

Hari Chana, MD, is a Family Physician using both acupuncture and Western medicine in his practice. He spends time in a senior's clinic one day per week and as a surgical assistant one day per week as a way to benefit his patients. He continues to take university courses in philosophy and topics that interest him.

Michael Enzle, PhD, is a Professor in the Department of Psychology at the University of Alberta, as well as Research Policy Coordinator in the Office of the Vice President of Research. His various research interests, including interpersonal relationships as well as moral judgment, made him a valuable and insightful member of the research team during the initial phase of the research.

Eric Higgs, PhD, is a Philosopher working in the areas of science, technology, and environment. He came to the University of Alberta in 1992 to work in the Departments of Philosophy, Anthropology, and Sociology with the Science, Technology, and Society Program. In January of 2002 he assumed the Directorship of the School of Environmental Studies at the University of Victoria, British Columbia.

Susan James, PhD, is Director of the Midwifery Education Program at Laurentian University in Sudbury, Ontario. She is a phenomenological researcher and collaborated with Ms. Briggs in the Phase II of the research in a subgroup looking at the ethical relationships between and among healthcare providers.

Helen Lantz, MHA, was the Chief Executive Officer for the Capital Care Group (a wholly owned subsidiary of the Capital

Health Authority) prior to her retirement in early 2002. Her practice has included public health nursing, teaching, and varying levels of healthcare administration. As the individual charged with the corporate responsibility for ethics from 1988 to 1997 (including chairing the ethics committee, policy development and ethics education), she was acutely aware of the ethical issues that professionals and nonprofessionals working in long-term care and assessment face in their practices.

Patricia Marck, RN, PhD, is an Assistant Professor in the Faculty of Nursing, University of Alberta, and an Adjunct Professor with the John Dossetor Health Ethics Centre. Currently, she is Professional Practice Leader—Nursing at the Royal Alexandra Hospital, Capital Health Authority. Her research program is aimed at investigating the theoretical and practical limits and strengths of an ecological, research-based approach to building and sustaining best practice environments.

Sandra McKinnon, RN, MN, now deceased, was an Oncology Nurse for many years and was Patient Care Manager of a Palliative Care Unit in a tertiary hospital, putting relational ethics into practice.

Bernie Pauly, RN, PhD(c), is currently a Doctoral Student in Nursing at the University of Victoria, British Columbia. Her focus of study is healthcare, policy, and ethics. As a participant in Phase I of the study, she was able to bring her practice experience and wisdom to the group in a way that spurred the project in new and meaningful directions.

David Schiff, MD, now deceased, was Director of a Neonatal Unit at a major tertiary hospital for many years and one of the original members of the Bioethics Project Steering Committee at the University of Alberta. His interest in ethics continued in his capacity as Acting Director in the Pediatric Ambulatory Services where he taught and practiced in the clinical setting in the ambulatory environment.

Margaret Shone, LLM, is Legal Counsel with the Alberta Law Reform Institute, has been instrumental in mental health reform in Canada, and was honored in Alberta for her contribution to human rights. She was a member of both phases of research and acted as a consultant to the Mental Health subgroup in Phase II. When not working, Ms. Shone is active in the acting community in Edmonton and the surrounding area.

Carl Urion, PhD, participated in Phase I of the project, prior to his retirement from the Department of Anthropology at the University of Alberta. His valuable insight came from not only his knowledge of linguistics but also from his native Cree heritage. In 2004, he received a national Aboriginal Achievement Award for a lifetime of education, research, and advocacy around native issues.

CONSULTANT TO THE RESEARCH PROJECT
Sally Gadow, PhD, is a Professor of Philosophy in the School of Nursing at the University of Colorado. We were fortunate to have Professor Gadow act as a consultant for the research project, especially during Phase I of the project. She shared her fine scholarship with the group along with her generous and gentle spirit.

Appendix B

Interdisciplinary Research Group Meetings

Meeting	Date	Program
1	19 June 1993	Introductory meeting
2	14 August 1993	Discuss readings by Raymond Duff, Edmund D. Pellegrino, and Sally Gadow
3	18 September 1993	View and discuss *Dax* video
4	30 October 1993	Further discussion of *Dax* video
5	27 November 1993	View and discuss *A Choice for K'aila* video
6	12 February 1994	Working paper no. 2 (yellow paper)
7	30 April 1994	View and discuss *Who Should Decide?* video and introduction of the images
8	18 June 1994	Visit by Sally Gadow
9	17 September 1994	Discussion of James's paper, "Letting Go of the Script"
10	3 December 1994	View *. . . And They Want a Child,* version 1
11	28 January 1995	Strawberry Creek retreat weekend
12	18 March 1995	Discussion of Marck's paper, "Outputs of the Retreat"
13	4 November 1995	Update from the various groups (video, slides, and workshop) and view video *. . . And They Want a Child,* version 2
14	26 and 27 June 1998	Weekend retreat
15	15 June 2001	Final meeting

Throughout the project, numerous analysis meetings took place that included investigators, members of the IRG, and students.

Made in the USA
Monee, IL
27 August 2022

12545216R10152